CHRIS JOHNSON'S

on target living
COOKING

eat healthy, feel satisfied, one delicious meal at a time

Written by Chris Johnson
with Bonnie Klinger

Design by CiesaDesign
Illustrations by Barbara Hranilovich

Published by

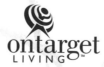

ontarget
LIVING™

On Target Living, Int'l
Haslett, Michigan

DEDICATION

For every person who is sick and tired of being sick and tired.

—Bonnie and Chris

ACKNOWLEDGMENTS

I want to thank my precious family and friends who have supported me, and the grumpy ogres who had the audacity to disagree with me during my life journey. Each one has challenged me to stretch my abilities to become all that I am now. I especially want to thank two people who taught me what I needed to know to write this cookbook. I met the first one 50 years ago and married him. He created the space in which I learned to love myself. I met the second two years ago and wrote a cookbook with him. He created *On Target Living* so I could learn to love my cells. Thanks, Jerry and Chris!

—Bonnie

Printed in the United States of America

Design: CiesaDesign, Lansing, Michigan
Illustrations: Barbara Hranilovich

WELCOME TO ON TARGET LIVING

This series of books is dedicated
to a healthy lifestyle.

ON TARGET LIVING COOKING

ON TARGET LIVING NUTRITION

DISCLAIMER

This publication contains the opinions and ideas of its authors.
Neither the publisher nor the authors are responsible for your
specific health or allergy needs that may require medical
supervision, or for any adverse reactions to the recipes contained in
this book. It is sold with the understanding that the authors and
publisher are not engaged in rendering medical, health, or any other
kind of personal professional services in the book. The reader should
consult his or her medical, health, or other competent professional
before adopting any of the suggestions in this book or drawing
inferences from it. The authors and publisher specifically disclaim
all responsibility for any liability, loss, or risk, personal or otherwise,
which is incurred as a consequence, directly or indirectly, of the use
and application of the contents of this book.

table of contents

Let's Get Cooking!

Breakfast

Snacks, Breads
and Beverages

Salads,
Dressings,
Dips, Sauces
and Seasonings

Soups and
Chilies

Entrées

Vegetables
and Sides

Desserts

Appendices

Index

INTRODUCTION

My life changed when I met Bonnie Klinger. Bonnie came to see me for a nutritional consultation with the single goal of losing weight. I knew I could help her meet that goal—and believed she would benefit beyond just losing weight in the process. At that first visit her eyes were lackluster, her energy low, and she had only enough hope to show up for the appointment her daughter made for her. I knew I could help her, and I did. What I didn't know was the impact Bonnie would have on my life. I already believed in the power of nutrition. I live it every day; in fact, I am a zealot about nurturing the body so it can heal itself. Yet, even to me—a true believer—the change I saw in Bonnie was incredible. Yes, Bonnie lost weight and improved her health, but the magic was in how her spirit was transformed. She developed a deep connection to her body and her health that can't be contained—when you see her, she glows. Bonnie showed me the power of the human spirit and taught me that no matter what your circumstances, or where you are in life, there is always hope. No matter what, you can make your life better.

I asked Bonnie to write a cookbook with me for one simple reason. She is a great cook, and I am not. Bonnie has developed hundreds of great tasting and healthy recipes following my *On Target Living Nutrition* principles, using the best ingredients for the best outcomes. This cookbook is unique in that it offers quality foods that taste great.

Bonnie changed her life and mine. Let her change yours.

Health & Happiness,
Chris Johnson

Chapter 1:
BONNIE'S JOURNEY

I have battled excess weight since I was a kid. I weighed 150 pounds when I was eleven years old, and my weight climbed to an all-time high of 207.6 pounds when I was in my late forties. I defined "healthy" as being thin! In high school, I started eating one meal a day to lose enough weight to make the cheerleading squad. I kept riding that insidious on-again off-again diet roller coaster for the next 45 years. I tried just about every diet—fasting, low-fat, high-fat, high-protein, low-carb, no-carb, good-carb-bad-carb, low-calorie and I even did the liquid meal replacement program. Besides being obese, I smoked two packs of cigarettes a day, seldom ate breakfast, ate lots of fast food, had a sedentary job, watched hours of television, and didn't do anything that could remotely be considered regular exercise. My spirit was nearly broken by all the failures.

Then to add insult to injury, my body went into malfunction mode (go figure!). I developed high blood pressure, hypothyroidism, osteoarthritis, allergies, high cholesterol, acid reflux, high triglycerides, low HDL, insulin resistance, and sleep apnea. At one time I was taking ten prescription medications plus aspirin each day. My cardiologist was planning to add even more medications and put me on a C-pap machine to aid my breathing while I slept. Yuck!

Through this entire struggle, I managed to lose twenty-nine pounds. Then I hit the dreaded, year-long plateau, despite diligently following a low-calorie diet and exercising three times a week. I was still taking eight prescription medications plus the aspirin. This was not my vision of retirement! When I realized I was giving my pharmacist enough money to count him as a dependent on my taxes, I knew things had to change.

What was missing?

Desperate people do desperate things, and I was desperate when I met with Chris Johnson in October of 2005. My daughter recommended that I make an appointment with Chris to learn more about nutrition, and boy, did I learn! Chris explained his On Target Living Nutrition program to me. I looked at his Food Target and thought to myself, "Oh boy, I'm in trouble. I don't like or eat fish, eggs, oatmeal, lentils, kale, flaxseeds and ostrich! Who eats ostrich?" My old ways of thinking about food and my focus on the negatives were big roadblocks for me. Chris said "I want you to be healthy at a cellular level." (What?) Throughout my life, my focus had been on reducing calories and losing weight! When Chris explained that my current way of eating was making me unhealthy at the cellular level and that was reflected in my current health profile, I finally got it! I was very skeptical about some changes Chris recommended, especially eating so often and eating more healthy fats. I thought, "Healthy fats, whoever heard that fats could be healthy?" My first thought was "I'm going to gain weight eating this way!" Chris said, "Give me six weeks and you will start feeling noticeably better!" Chris also said that by getting healthier at the cellular level and working with my physician, I could likely wean myself off some of my medications by the end of the year. So I thought, "Well, why not? Nothing else has worked so far."

So, at the age of sixty-two, I started my journey to a healthier me! I went home and cleaned out my cupboards, refrigerator and freezer of all processed foods. If the label said "partially-hydrogenated or high-fructose corn syrup," out it went. I went to three health food stores and restocked my pantry with flaxseed oil, cod liver oil, evening primrose oil, extra virgin olive oil, extra virgin coconut oil, rolled oats, venison, buffalo, organic dairy, organic chicken, fresh fruits and vegetables. My husband and I prepared all of our home meals and snacks from these new foods and made even healthier choices in restaurants. I worked with my personal trainer and daughter Rebecca Klinger, who added several "interval" workouts to my cardio routine along with my current three sessions of strength training per week. I described what I was doing to my family physician and enlisted her support, as Chris suggested. My physician encouraged me to keep track of my blood pressure and have blood work done after several weeks to monitor my response to the exercise and nutritional changes.

After only nine weeks of *On Target Living Nutrition*, I had lost seventeen pounds. That was more than I had lost in any of the previous four years! My blood pressure, cholesterol and triglycerides had improved so dramatically that my physician discontinued six medications and the daily aspirin. My cholesterol and triglycerides were better than they were when I was taking 10mg of a popular statin drug. Suddenly, instead of building a new wing on my local pharmacy, I was living like a "normal person."

What is significant for me is that from the time I started *On Target Living Nutrition* until the end of the 9-week period, the only thing that changed was what and how often I ate. Other than the additional interval training, my exercise, sleep patterns and water consumption remained consistent.

I now define "healthy" as having cells that function the way they were designed to. And, surprise, surprise, having healthy cells has led to a healthier weight! I am eating foods that taste, smell and look delicious and are easy to prepare. I have eliminated artificial sweeteners, most added refined sugar, high fructose corn syrup, and trans fats. I have replaced refined or processed foods with whole foods. I have added healthy fats to bring out the flavor of the food and provide hunger satiety, a first for me! I eat proteins that contain less saturated fat— chicken breast, fish, beans, wild game, and buffalo. I eat many more servings of fresh or frozen fruits and vegetables and have switched to whole grains. I still occasionally eat processed foods or foods that contain sugar or white flour—restaurant pizza or a favorite holiday dessert or a small piece of candy. However, at least 95 percent of my food appears on the three inner circles of the Food Target.

What's so different about *On Target Living Nutrition?*

On other weight loss plans I would get one or two results—short-term weight loss, better cholesterol numbers OR lower blood pressure, then back on the roller coaster.

On Target Living Nutrition delivered:

- Weight loss/weight control!
- Improved cholesterol and blood lipids!
- Improved blood pressure!
- Improved physical and mental energy!
- Improved satiety—I never have that gnawing hunger I experienced on every other weight loss plan!
- Fewer prescription medications—only two instead of ten!
- Sustainability—I have maintained these changes for over a year, so I consider them a lifestyle change!

Achieving these results is like winning an Olympic gold medal, the Kentucky Derby and a Super Bowl ring, all rolled into one! Losing more than fifty-five pounds, regaining my health, feeling physically stronger and younger, buying a new size ten wardrobe and throwing away bottles and bottles of prescription medications have been incredibly rewarding.

But wait! There's more! The most profound outcome is the remarkable mental and emotional transformation I continue to experience. For the first time in my life, I feel like the person I am meant to be. The next part of my journey will contain so much more joy, health and happiness because I took the huge, scary steps that were necessary. I moved away from mindless eating (my feeble attempt to satisfy my mouth and emotional hunger) and moved toward mindful eating that nourished my cells. I reclaimed my life, and regained a sense of personal power that I can do something so loving to and for myself.

On Target Living Nutrition exists because of Chris Johnson's knowledge, compassion and dedication to help others find their optimal health. I want to thank him again for being who he is and for his continued support.

Left: Bonnie before making healthy choices. Right: Bonnie today

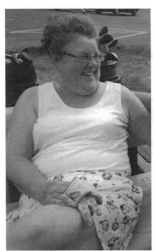
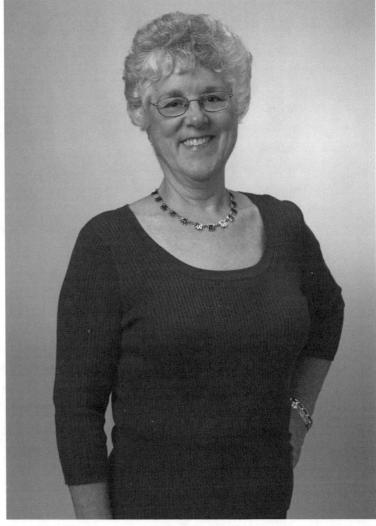

Chapter 2
WHY WRITE A COOKBOOK?

As I was applying the *On Target Living Nutrition* concepts to my cooking, I discovered that none of my old recipes fit very well into my new way of eating. Most of the recipes in my older cookbooks exclusively used the "whites"—white sugar, white flour, white rice, white potatoes. I kept modifying my old recipes and developing new recipes.

I reviewed many cookbooks that emphasized healthy eating. These books focused mostly on weight loss or decreasing heart disease, type 2 diabetes, or insulin resistance. Some of these supported low-fat diets, others focused on eating any fat and protein, but drastically reducing all carbohydrates. Many times they classified "good" versus "bad" carbohydrates based solely on the glycemic index! Some cookbooks replace sugar with artificial sweeteners, promote lower salt intake or lower fat intake or encourage eating whole and even all-raw foods. Several of the newer books have two or three levels of eating: 1) a detoxification phase, 2) a weight loss phase, and/or 3) a lifestyle maintenance stage. They even include passing references to the importance of managing stress, drinking sufficient amounts of water, including healthier fats and getting enough sleep and exercise. But even in the more moderate approaches, "fat phobia" prevails. Many of these books fail to emphasize that some fats actually help your body function more effectively. They certainly don't make precise recommendations for how and in what quantity to incorporate these healthy fats into your diet.

I know that no one system of cooking and eating is right for everyone, but I believe that most people will have more physical and mental energy, be healthier and lead a happier life if they feed the cells in their body what they need to work at their optimum level. I went from being sluggish and prescription-dependent to being healthy and full of energy! The price of admission to this party is that I have to pay attention to the quality of the foods I eat and to maintain other lifestyle changes—no smoking, plenty of exercise, water, sleep, and stress management.

This is not a diet cookbook in the sense that eating this way is only for people who want to lose weight. Being thin does not automatically mean you are healthy. You don't need to have multiple medical diagnoses, be severally medicated, or be overweight for *On Target Living Nutrition* to improve your health and life. The increased energy that occurs when you feed your cells high quality nutrients is worth all the time and effort it takes to make these changes.

Chapter 3
REGAIN YOUR SENSE OF PERSONAL POWER

My exercise, food and thinking patterns have changed slowly over the past forty-five years. That is due, in part, to my readiness and willingness to do the hard work of change, but also because updated information about the positive and negative impacts of food, exercise, sleep deprivation and stress on our bodies is just now exploding into the media.

If you want to improve your body's health at the cellular level, and you are ready to make some big or small nutritional changes, try some of these recipes. Change the ingredients to fit your tastes. Experiment with herbs and spices. But whatever you do, **CHANGE**. Change **something** that will improve your life and health. I made major changes to my nutritional program, literally overnight! I was desperate, I knew I had to change and I was willing to do whatever it took to get my life back! I realize that you may not be ready to eliminate sugar or eat wild game meats or prepare most of your meals at home.

Even if you are not ready to make many changes quickly, you could drink more water, add the healthy fats to your daily eating, make one pot of soup a week to get more vegetables, move your body more, pack a healthy lunch, or read food labels—any of these changes will get you on the path to healthier cells. I want you to become your healthiest! I want you to enjoy the food you eat! Most of all, I want you to regain your sense of personal power!

Chapter 4
WHAT MAKES ON TARGET LIVING COOKING UNIQUE?

So how are these recipes different from those found in other "healthy" cookbooks?

These recipes were developed by Chris Johnson and me from the concepts outlined in Chris's *On Target Living Nutrition* book, and further illustrated in Chris's *On Target Living* seminars. Every recipe—yes, even the ostrich soup—was tested in my kitchen. All of these recipes call for ingredients that pack the maximum amount of nutrients (quality) into the minimum amount of calories (quantity), while keeping the taste, texture and appearance satisfying. That is a pretty tall order for some little unsuspecting ingredients—to give your body "good stuff" and eliminate "bad stuff," to replace neutral or unhealthy ingredients that fail to give your body any nutrition (or, worse yet, give your body products that makes it function poorly) with ingredients that have their nutritional components intact and to help your body function as it was meant to.

How are these recipes unique?

The primary difference is how the ingredients are raised and processed before they get to you. Many of the ingredients may sound familiar. There may also be some ingredients— ground flaxseeds, ostrich, buffalo, soy products—with which you may be unfamiliar. Each of these ingredients is chosen to improve the nutritional quality of what you eat, to replace the unhealthy fats with healthy fats, and to replace refined, highly-processed foods with unprocessed, whole foods.

What are *quality* ingredients?

Wild-caught fish, organic meats, organic dairy, fruits, vegetables, whole grains, spices, and seasonings were used to develop and test these recipes, whenever available. If an organic product was not available, then "natural" products were used. If a "natural" product was not available, then a conventionally grown product was used. Feel free to use the level with which you are most comfortable. Just remember that you will receive the greatest nutritional benefit if you use organic ingredients.

"Why would I want to waste time and money looking for organic sources of my food," you ask? The short answer is to decrease the amount of food additives, pesticides, hormones, antibiotics, and chemicals that you would otherwise eat in conventionally-grown and conventionally-processed food!

Organic foods grown and processed in the United States and imported from abroad must meet a rigorous certification process monitored by the United States Department of Agriculture. The use of synthetic fertilizers, toxic and persistent pesticides, irradiation, sewage sludge or gene modification is NOT permitted at any time during growing or processing. Organic foods cannot contain artificial flavors, colors, or preservatives.

"Natural" foods typically advertise that they exclude artificial flavors, colors and preservatives, but may use artificial fertilizers, synthetic pesticides, irradiation and gene modification in the growing process. The labels on the "natural" foods may also indicate that the product was grown without antibiotics, hormones and steroids. However, these claims on natural foods offer no protection as they are not monitored by any certification process.

In conventionally-grown and processed products, antibiotics, hormones, steroids, synthetic pesticides, irradiation and gene modification, as well as artificial flavors, colors, preservatives and fertilizers, are all allowed.

Carbohydrates

GRAINS, FRUIT, VEGETABLES

Whole grains contain oil. Once the whole grain is ground, as in whole grain flour, the flour can get rancid as it ages. For that reason, buy your organic whole grain flours from a store that has a good turnover. Keep your whole grain flours in tightly sealed containers in the refrigerator or freezer (a zip-lock bag works very nicely).

The most recently picked organic fruits and vegetables have the most nutrients. Frozen organic fruits and vegetables are generally comparable to fresh. Sometimes, the only option is organic canned.

The plant-based ingredients agar powder, arrowroot, and stevia have been substituted for gelatin, cornstarch and granulated sugar/artificial sweeteners in these recipes. Each of these ingredients has more health benefits and is less processed than the conventional options.

Agar is a plant-based starch that can be used as an alternative to animal-based gelatin. Agar is obtained from red marine algae that can be used as a gelling agent. Use one-half teaspoon of fine agar powder to gel one cup of liquid. Bring the liquid to a boil; add the agar and simmer for one minute. Amazingly, the agar will gel the liquid without refrigeration.

Arrowroot is a plant-based starch that can be used as an alternative to highly-refined cornstarch. Arrowroot powder is produced from the dried arrowroot plant. It makes an excellent thickener for Asian stir-fry, soups and gravies. Substitute two teaspoons of arrowroot for one tablespoon of cornstarch or for one and one-half tablespoons of flour. Dissolve two teaspoons of arrowroot in two tablespoons of cold water and add to your recipe. Do not over stir, as the arrowroot will begin to lose its thickening properties.

Stevia is a green, leafy herb that is up to 300 times sweeter than granulated sugar. It has no calories and does not impact blood sugar levels. The benefit of using stevia is that it eliminates artificial sweeteners and decreases the use of white sugar. Stevia is available in leaf, liquid extract and powder forms. You will get a wide-range of results depending on the particular form you use. To get more consistency, Stevia Plus™, a powdered blend, has been used in all these recipes. (Refer to the Appendix on Herbs and Spices [p 219] for more information on stevia.) To substitute Stevia Plus™ for granulated sugar, use a one-to-four ratio. For example, one-fourth teaspoon Stevia Plus™ equals one teaspoon granulated sugar; one tablespoon Stevia Plus™ equals one-qurter cup granulated sugar, etc.

There is a slight aftertaste with stevia, but this is improved by adding vanilla or maple extract to the recipe. When beginning to use stevia in a recipe, replace half of the granulated sugar or artificial sweetener with stevia; then gradually decrease the sugar or artificial sweetener, and increase the stevia proportionally. I still use a small amount of granulated sugar in most recipes for taste. If you are not ready to use stevia in the recipes, replace the stevia with organic sugar, using the 1 to 4 ratio. If using sugar, increase the nutritional values for total calories and carbohydrates, 208 calories and 52 carbohydrates for every quarter cup.

The bottom line is that many foods give our bodies and cells the powerful nutrients our cells need to function. Some foods just give us empty calories per serving, and some foods actually harm our cells. The guidelines in these recipes direct you to the healthiest foods.

So where do you find these new ingredients? More and more grocery stores, especially the larger chains, now carry a wide assortment of organic foods. Health food stores, especially in bigger cities, carry most of these products or can advise you of a source.

Please note: Many of the recipes make one to two servings, and several of the soup recipes make five to six cups, to encourage people in smaller households to cook for themselves. These recipes are easily doubled or tripled for larger households.

Proteins

MEATS, FISH, DAIRY

If you can only afford or find organic products in one macronutrient category, I strongly recommend that you spend the extra time and money to locate and buy organic meats, dairy, eggs and wild-caught fish. These products are at the top of the food chain. Therefore, conventionally-grown animals carry the heaviest concentrations of antibiotics, hormones, steroids, toxic and persistent pesticides and synthetic fertilizers because the foods they eat have also been grown on soil to which toxic and persistent pesticides and synthetic fertilizers have been applied.

Many recipes use meats that may be new to you—venison, ostrich or buffalo. These meats are significantly lower in calories and 50 to 75 percent lower in saturated fat than similar cuts of beef. However, if you are not ready to try these meats or they are not available, just substitute organic ground turkey, flank steak or ground round. Be sure you increase the nutritional values for total calories and fat, if beef is used.

Fats

OILS, NUTS, SEEDS

All the oils used in these recipes are organic, unrefined, expeller pressed oils, to eliminate the chemicals used to grow, extract and refine conventionally-produced oils. Another unique feature of unrefined oils is that their nutrients are left intact. Conventionally-produced oils are stripped of their nutrition when they are heated and chemicals are added. The oils used in most of these recipes are extra virgin olive oil, extra virgin coconut oil, almond oil, macadamia nut oil, or expeller pressed canola oil. Extra virgin coconut oil, almond oil, macadamia nut oil and expeller pressed canola oil can be used in high-temperature cooking without damaging their nutritional values. Extra virgin olive oil maintains maximum health benefits and flavor if used unheated or at lower temperatures—325° or less. Each of the oils, except expeller pressed canola oil, has a wonderful flavor and aroma that contributes to the nutrition and taste of the recipe. Because expeller pressed canola oil does not have a strong flavor, I use it in some dessert recipes so the sweet spices aren't overpowered by the competing flavor of the oil. Some of the uncooked recipes include flaxseed oil, which should not be heated. Ground flaxseeds can be added to recipes that will be heated or baked, because heating will not reduce their health benefits.

Whenever possible, buy raw nuts and seeds for the same reason you use unrefined oils— the blanching process reduces the nutritional values.

Equipment used

There are hundreds of pots, pans, utensils, small and large appliances and gadgets on the market to help the home cook. A list of kitchen equipment that was used to make these recipes is included in the Appendix. Inventory your kitchen and add what you need for the recipes you want to try.

Ingredients used

On Target Living Nutrition offers an amazing variety of fruits, vegetables, meats, grains and seasonings. All the ingredients that have been used to test these recipes are included in a shopping list in the Appendix. Make copies of the shopping list to help you inventory your pantry, then take it to the store to stock up or just get ingredients for a particular recipe.

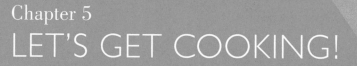

Chapter 5
LET'S GET COOKING!

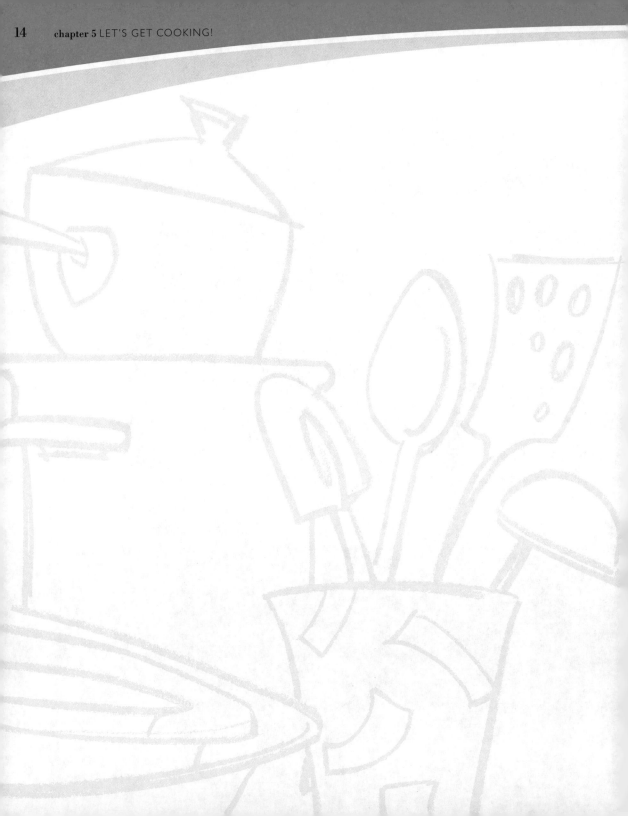

Chapter 5
LET'S GET COOKING!

Do you have one or two hours available every night to prepare meals? No? Me, either! But the fact is that cooking with whole foods at home takes more time than cooking with pre-packaged, processed foods, grabbing some take-out, or eating in a restaurant. It takes forethought and planning. Here are the steps I use:

1. **Pick a recipe.** Many of the recipes can be made ahead for use later in the week or frozen for a later meal. See the table on page 16 for some ideas. Eventually, develop a menu plan for several meals for each week and go through the same steps.

2. **Inventory your kitchen.** Check the kitchen to be sure you have the necessary pans and tools. (See Appendix [p 213] for suggested equipment.)

3. **Buy the food.** At first, this took me the most time. Because I decided to eat organic foods, I had to learn about organic food and then locate the stores and products in those stores that I wanted to use. In addition, many of the brands I had used for years no longer fit in my eating plan because I eliminated trans fats, high fructose corn syrup, artificial flavorings and those words none of us can pronounce. So, a sub-step here may be for you to locate your new food sources and brands.

4. **Make the recipe.** Many of the recipes have times listed for cooking, so you can plan when the meal will be completed.

5. **Eat the food.** This is the best part! Be sure to take your time and savor these foods.

6. **Start getting healthier cells with every bite!** You don't even have to schedule any time for this part. Once you have fed your cells with healthy food, those little rascals will do this part all on their own.

Your other option is to:

1. Buy food of unknown origin and quality at a restaurant or make a quick meal using some highly-processed foods with most of the nutrients stripped away.

2. Eat the food.

3. Continue the eating habits that are keeping your cells sick!

I don't want to be harsh, but I believe this is the choice each of us makes whenever we eat: Do I want this meal to make my cells healthier? Or, am I just too busy to care what this food will do to my body?

The following table gives some time-saving tips to help you include healthier eating in your day.

TIME SAVING TIPS

MEAL	TIME-SAVING TIPS
Breakfast	• *Oatmeal On-The-Run* (p 25) for the next day's breakfast • *Creamy Oatmeal* (p 25) for next day's breakfast; make extra servings and warm up as needed.
Snack at Work	• *Parfait On-the-Run* (p 28) • See *Quick Balanced Snacks* (p 43)
Lunch at Work	• Toss your choices from *Salad Bar in a Bag* (p 63) into a zip-top bag; pour your salad dressing of choice into a small container and put both in an insulated lunch bag. • Take any of your purposefully created leftovers (see below). • Take leftover soup in a thermos or warm it up at work
Lunch at Home	• Make one soup each week, so there are leftovers for lunch. Many of the soups freeze very well. • Use any of your purposefully created leftovers (see below).
Lunch/Dinner	**Purposefully create leftovers with double or triple batches. Cooked, tightly-covered food will typically be safe to eat for three days in your refrigerator. Foods stored in zip top bags or plastic containers can be frozen for up to three months and still maintain their quality (be sure to label these with contents and dates). When you are ready to use the frozen food, put it in the refrigerator the night before you plan to eat it or in a sink full of cold water for an hour so it will thaw, then proceed with your recipe.** • *Basic Meat Sauce:* divide it into 2-cup portions and freeze in zip top bags to be used in Sloppy Joes, Too, Sauce for Spaghetti or Lasagna, Spanish Rice, Goulash, Autumn Soup, Fast Chili, Southwestern Bean Soup, or Taco Salad. • *Sauce for Spaghetti or Lasagna:* divide it into 2-cup portions and freeze in zip top bags to be used in Zucchini Pasta, Zucchini Lasagna, Spaghetti with Sauce, or Spaghetti Squash Spaghetti. • *Steamed Rice:* freeze the extra portion in a zip top bag to steam later or make Basic Fried Rice. • *Salad Bar in a Bag:* use for salad, fried rice, quiche, frittata, stir-fry, soup, or roasting. • Leftover *Roasted Vegetables:* Pita Pizza, Stuffed Pita, add to salads or scrambled eggs, replace vegetables in quiche or frittata recipes or toss into soups at the end of cooking. • Leftover cooked chicken: Chicken Salad for sandwiches, Chicken Fried Rice, Chicken Waldorf Salad, Chicken Caesar Salad, Nancy's Mexican Soup, or White Chicken Chili. • Leftover cooked salmon: salads or Salmon Asparagus Soup.

You may already have a collection of recipes that you and your family enjoy. So, do you just throw them out and start all over? No! Here are a few general suggestions that may help you make your favorite recipes healthier.

HOW TO MAKE YOUR OLD FAVORITES HEALTHY

Type of Recipe	HOW TO MAKE YOUR OLD FAVORITES HEALTHIER
All recipes	Replace the unhealthy fats with unrefined extra virgin olive oil, extra virgin coconut oil, macadamia nut oil, or almond oil.
Burgers, meatloaf	• Replace half of the ground beef or pork with an equal amount of ground all white meat turkey. • Add ½ cup of cooked and mashed beans or lentils to the burger mixture to increase the fiber content.
Soups	Double the vegetables.
Salads	• Use Romaine lettuce or spinach instead of iceberg lettuce. • Use dressings made with extra virgin olive oil.
Pasta dishes	• Replace half of the full-fat cheese with low-fat cheese. • Use whole grain pasta instead of white. To adjust to the different taste and texture, begin by replacing one-fourth of the white pasta with an equal amount of whole grain pasta. Then gradually increase the amount of whole grain pasta in the recipe, until you are using all whole grain. • Sauté one cup of onions, mushrooms, broccoli or a couple of handfuls of spinach in one tablespoon of extra virgin olive oil, and then add prepared spaghetti sauce to top your whole grain pasta.
Casseroles	• Add more vegetables. • Replace white flour noodles with whole grain noodles. • Replace white potatoes with sweet, blue or redskin potatoes.
Sandwiches	• Switch to whole grain breads, tortillas, and pitas. • Pile on the vegetables (tomatoes, Romaine, onion, salsa, cucumber, etc.).
Muffins, breads	• Replace one-third of the white flour with whole grain flour; evaluate the result, and continue to increase the proportion of whole grain flour to maintain your satisfaction with the result. • Add fruit—blueberries, raisins, chopped apples (unpeeled). • Replace ¼ cup of the flour with the equivalent amount of ground flaxseeds.
Desserts	Replace one-fourth of the white sugar in a recipe with the equivalent amount of Stevia Plus™ blend; evaluate the result, and continue to increase the proportion of Stevia Plus™ to maintain your satisfaction with the result.

Information for calories and grams of carbohydrates (CHO), total FAT, protein (PRO) and dietary fiber are provided for each recipe. Nutrition information was calculated using product information from manufacturers and listings in *The Complete Book of Food Counts* by Corinne T. Netzer (6th edition, Dell, 2003). If total grams for an ingredient or the whole recipe equaled .4 or less, the gram count was rounded down to the nearest whole number; if it was .5 or more, it was rounded up to the nearest whole number. Information is given per serving or a specific measured quantity. Information is calculated on the first measurement of the first ingredient listed. If a range is given (½ to ⅔ cup rolled oats, for example), information is calculated on the ½ cup amount. Optional ingredients or second or third choices of ingredients are not included in the nutritional information. For example, several recipes list beef as the first meat choice.

The nutritional information was figured using the values for beef. If buffalo, chicken, turkey or venison is used to replace the beef, the total calories for the recipe will be fewer, and saturated fat will be reduced by 50 percent or more.

But what do you do if there's an ingredient you don't like, have an allergy to or is not available? Do you just not make that recipe? No! Substitute. Use what works for you. These recipes are meant to be guidelines, a way for you to begin to evaluate what you eat and to add healthier foods that you enjoy. Some ingredients are listed with the brand name product used to develop these recipes, so you get the same results when you make the recipe. Refer to the table below for options.

The ingredients listed in the **Instead of** column are those used in the development and testing of these recipes. The ingredients listed in the **Use** column are options you may want to choose. Be aware that you may have to adapt the recipe (cooking time, amount of liquid, etc.) if you make substitutions, and it will have a taste and texture that is different from the original. (Just between you and me, I almost never make a recipe the same way two times in a row.)

I have marked my favorites in each recipe category with a 🌺. These recipes rank as favorites because they are tasty AND easy to prepare.

Have fun!

KEY FOR INGREDIENT SUBSTITUTION

Instead of:	Use:
2 cups *Basic Meat Sauce*	8 ounces ground turkey, ground venison, or ground round, plus 8 ounces tomato sauce, ½ cup chopped onion, ¼ cup chopped green pepper, 1 clove minced garlic, and 1 teaspoon Italian seasoning
Ground buffalo	Ground turkey, ground ostrich, ground venison, ground round, soy "meat" substitute
Cow's milk	Almond milk, goat milk, oat milk, rice milk, soy milk,
Dairy cheeses	soy cheeses, goat cheese
Whey protein powder	Rice, soy, hemp protein powder or goatein protein powder
Whole wheat flour	Brown rice, kamut, buckwheat, spelt, or rye flour—just be sure the label says whole grain as the first ingredient
Whole wheat pasta	Brown rice, sprouted whole grain (wheat, spelt, barley, millet, lentil, soybean), kamut, kamut and buckwheat, spelt, rye, quinoa, rice/potato/soy pasta—just be sure the label says whole grain
Whole wheat bread	Any whole grain or sprouted grain bread (see whole wheat pasta, above)
Red-skin potato	Sweet potato, blue/purple potato
Raisins	Dried apples, apricots, blueberries, cherries, cranberries
Red raspberries	Apple, blackberries, blueberries, peaches, strawberries,
Extra virgin olive oil	Extra virgin coconut oil, almond oil, macadamia nut oil, all unrefined
Canola mayonnaise	Light canola mayonnaise
Almonds	Almond butter, pecans, pine nuts, walnuts, ground flaxseeds (flaxseed oil can be substituted, but ONLY in uncooked recipes)
1 tablespoon sugar ¼ cup sugar	1 tablespoon honey or ¾ teaspoon Stevia Plus™ ¼ cup honey or 1 tablespoon Stevia Plus™

Chapter 6
RECIPES

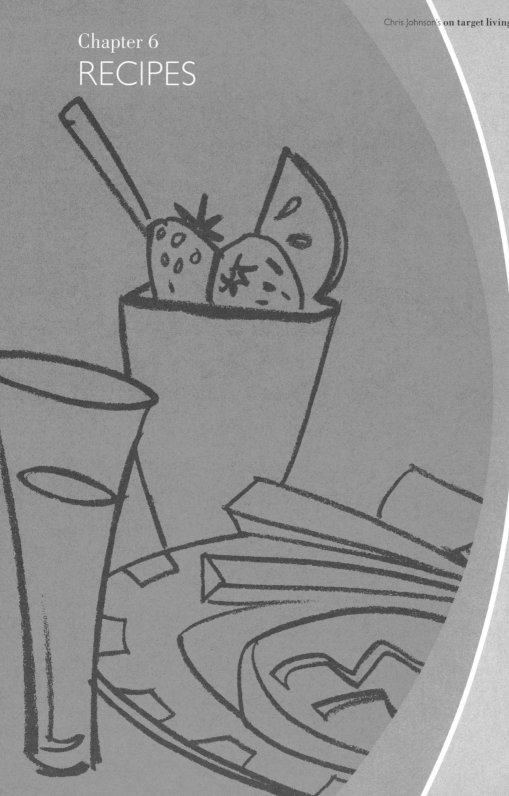

recipes

BREAKFAST

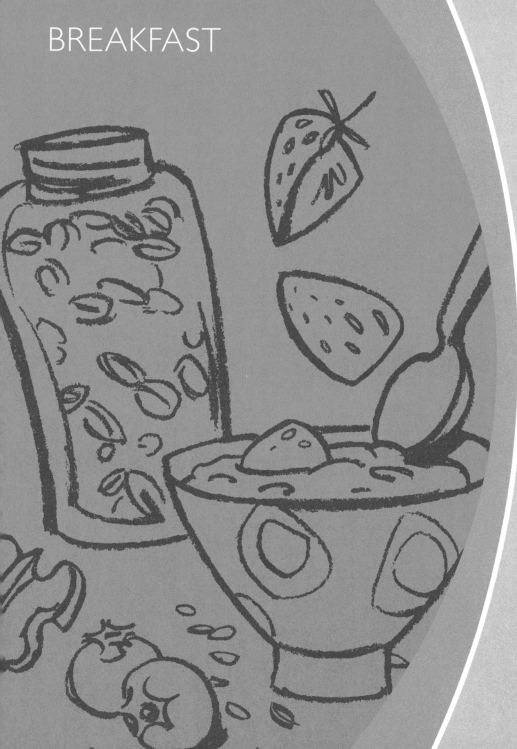

breakfast

 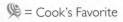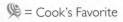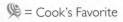
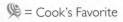 = Cook's Favorite

blender breakfast

Serves 2
352 Calories per serving; 33g CHO; 16g FAT; 19g PRO; 6g Fiber

½   cup soy milk
6   ounces firm tofu
1   scoop soy protein powder
2   cups frozen fruit
3   tablespoons flaxseed oil
1   banana
1   teaspoon vanilla extract
¼   teaspoon Stevia Plus™ blend (optional)

Combine all ingredients in blender and mix until smooth.

breakfast sandwich

Serves 1
245 Calories per serving; 35g CHO; 9g FAT; 8g PRO; 5g Fiber

1   slice whole wheat toast
1   tablespoon natural peanut butter
½   banana, sliced

Spread the peanut butter on the toast; top with sliced banana. Serve with a glass of milk.

breakfast burrito

Serves I
276 Calories per serving; 28g CHO; 12g FAT; 14g PRO; 7g Fiber

| 8-inch whole wheat or sprouted grain tortilla
| teaspoon extra virgin olive oil
¼ cup onion
¼ cup broccoli slaw
| whole egg + I egg white (free-range, beaten)
  sea salt and freshly-ground black pepper, to taste
2 tablespoons salsa

In a small skillet, heat olive oil over low heat; sauté vegetables for 2 minutes.
Add eggs, salt and pepper and scramble. Warm tortilla for 10 seconds in
microwave, if desired. Spread egg mixture across center of tortilla; top with salsa.
Fold up bottom, then each side to form a pocket.

CJ's oatmeal on-the-run (cold, uncooked)

Serves I
526 Calories per serving; 47g CHO; 29g FAT; 13g PRO 10g Fiber

½ cup rolled oats
1½ tablespoons fresh or frozen fruit
| tablespoon slivered almonds
2 teaspoons lemon-flavored cod liver oil
| tablespoon flaxseed oil
½ cup soy milk or organic skim milk
| dash ground cinnamon

Place all ingredients in a small bowl with lid. Let stand in refrigerator overnight
or for 10 minutes prior to eating. No cooking required. Fast, easy, healthy and
tastes great!

oatmeal on-the-run (cold, uncooked)

Serves 1
336 Calories per serving; 47g CHO; 10g FAT; 13g PRO; 10g Fiber

½   cup rolled oats
1½ tablespoons fruit
 1 tablespoons slivered almonds
½   cup soy milk or organic skim milk

Place all ingredients in a small bowl with lid. Let stand in refrigerator overnight
or for 10 minutes prior to eating. No cooking required. Fast, easy, healthy and
tastes great.

creamy oatmeal (hot, cooked)

Serves 1
342 Calories per serving; 59g CHO; 7g FAT; 14g PRO; 9g Fiber

¼   cup rolled oats
⅔   cup skim milk
 1 tablespoon dried fruit
¼   cup natural unsweetened applesauce
½   teaspoon Stevia Plus™ blend
 2 drops vanilla extract
¼   teaspoon cinnamon
    Dash of sea salt
 1 tablespoon ground flaxseeds

Put all ingredients, except ground flaxseeds, into a small saucepan; cover and
refrigerate overnight. When ready to serve, heat over medium heat just to boiling;
reduce heat and simmer for 7 minutes, stirring occasionally. Pour into bowl;
sprinkle with ground flaxseeds. Double or triple this recipe for "purposefully
created leftovers." Store leftovers in the refrigerator for up to four days.

oatmeal plus (hot or cold)

Serves 1
388 Calories per serving, 48g CHO; 12g FAT; 22g PRO; 11g Fiber

1¼	cups water
½	scoop soy or rice protein powder
⅔	cup rolled oats
1	teaspoon cinnamon
1½	tablespoons dried fruit
1	tablespoon walnuts, almonds, ground flaxseeds or flaxseed oil
1	teaspoon vanilla extract
½	cup soy milk or organic skim milk

In a saucepan, mix water and protein powder well. Add oats and bring to a boil, stirring occasionally. When mixture starts to thicken, cover and turn off the heat. Let stand for 10 minutes and add the remaining ingredients. Mix well and serve.

heart healthy granola

7 cups
½ cup = 292 Calories; 47g CHO; 8g FAT; 8g PRO (excluding milk); 7g Fiber

6	cups rolled oats
2	tablespoons almond oil
⅓	cup ground flaxseeds
2	tablespoons brown sugar
1	cup dried fruit
1½	cups dried apples, chopped into small pieces

Preheat oven to 350°. Mix all ingredients, except dried fruit, in a large bowl. Spread evenly in a shallow baking pan and bake for 15 minutes. Remove from oven and stir, so granola will cook uniformly. Bake an additional 10-15 minutes until golden. Remove from oven and mix in dried fruit. Cool and store in a covered container. Add ½ cup milk to granola when serving (optional). Your kids will love this for breakfast and snacks.

CJ's granola

13 cups
¼ cup = 102 Calories; 16g CHO; 3g FAT; 3g PRO; 3g Fiber

 6   tablespoons water
 2   teaspoons Stevia Plus™ blend
 3   tablespoons extra virgin coconut oil, melted
 ½   teaspoon sea salt
 1   tablespoon vanilla extract
 9   cups rolled oats
 ¾   cup raw, sliced almonds and sunflower seeds
 ½   cup ground flaxseeds
 1   tablespoon cinnamon
 ½   teaspoon ground nutmeg
2¼   cups chopped dried apples
 ¾   cup chopped prunes

Preheat oven to 275°. In small bowl, mix water, Stevia Plus™, coconut oil, salt, and vanilla; set aside. In large bowl, mix oats, almonds, ground flaxseeds, cinnamon, and nutmeg. Pour water mixture over oats mixture. Stir to blend thoroughly. Spread on cookie sheet. Bake 45-60 minutes, stirring two times. Remove from oven and cool thoroughly. Add dried fruits. Refrigerate to keep flaxseeds fresh. Use in *Parfait On-The-Run* (p 28), as a cold cereal with milk, as a cooked cereal (½ cup granola cooked for 7 minutes with ¾ to 1 cup water), or as a snack.

🌹 parfait on-the-run

Serves 1
393 Calories per serving; 41g CHO; 21g FAT; 8g PRO; 10g Fiber

½   cup frozen blueberries
½   cup low-fat yogurt, any flavor
¼   cup *CJ's Granola* (p 27)
3   tablespoons ground flaxseeds

Layer ingredients in order given in a 2-cup plastic covered container. Cover container and put in insulated lunch bag with small ice pack. Toss in a spoon. When it's time for breakfast, mid-morning or mid-afternoon snack, stir the contents up and enjoy. (Can be made the night before and refrigerated.)

yogurt crunch

Serves 2
201 Calories per serving; 28g CHO; 5g FAT; 11g PRO; 6g Fiber

1   cup non-fat plain or vanilla yogurt
1   packet Stevia Plus™
¾   cup fresh blueberries
¼   cup rolled oats
2   tablespoons slivered or slicedalmonds
    dash of cinnamon

Spoon yogurt into bowl and add Stevia Plus™, if desired. Add fruit and nuts, top with rolled oats and sprinkle with cinnamon. Eat immediately or store in refrigerator. Great for breakfast, lunch or as a snack.

egg white omelet

Serves 2
196 Calories per serving; 5g CHO; 12g FAT; 17g PRO; 1g Fiber (excluding the fruit)

½   tablespoon extra virgin olive oil
¼   cup sliced or chopped onion
¼   cup sliced or chopped green or red bell pepper
¼   cup sliced or chopped mushrooms (approximately 6)
4   egg whites (free-range)
2   whole eggs (free-range)
1   tablespoon shredded low-fat cheddar cheese

Heat half the oil in an omelet pan or skillet, sauté vegetables; remove from pan; set aside. Heat the remaining oil in the pan. Pour beaten eggs into skillet. As eggs begin to set, lift edges and tilt pan to move uncooked eggs to bottom. Spread cooked vegetables over half the eggs. Sprinkle on cheese. Flip remaining half of eggs over vegetables and cheese. Serve with sliced fruit.

CJ's 3-minute scrambled eggs

Serves 1
256 Calories per serving; 2g CHO; 14g FAT; 26g PRO; 0g Fiber

1   teaspoon extra virgin coconut oil
4   egg whites (free-range)
2   whole eggs (free-range)

Heat oil in a medium skillet over medium heat. Add egg whites and whole eggs and stir with a fork. Scramble until cooked.

scrambled eggs

Serves 2
230 Calories per serving; 10g CHO; 14g FAT; 16g PRO; 3g Fiber

2   egg whites (free-range)
2   whole eggs (free-range)
1   large garlic clove, minced
1   tablespoon chopped fresh oregano
½   red bell pepper, diced
½   green bell pepper, diced
½   small white onion, diced
½   tablespoon extra virgin olive oil
    sea salt and freshly-ground black pepper, to taste
1   tablespoon grated low-fat cheddar or swiss cheese

Whisk eggs and herbs in medium bowl. Stir in peppers and onion. Lightly coat
a medium skillet with olive oil and heat over medium heat. Pour egg mixture
into skillet. Add garlic, oregano, salt and pepper; scramble until cooked. Sprinkle
with cheddar or swiss cheese.

simple seafood scramble

Serves 2
221 Calories per serving; 6g CHO; 13g FAT; 20g PRO; 2g Fiber

4 egg whites (free-range)
2 whole eggs (free-range)
1 tablespoon fchopped resh basil
1 teaspoon chopped fresh dill
½ cup chopped cooked shrimp, crab or scallops (or combination)
1 tablespoon extra virgin olive oil
1 large garlic clove, pressed
1 stalk celery, minced
¼ cup finely-chopped tomato
2 scallions, finely chopped
¼ cup finely-chopped mushrooms
   sea salt and freshly-ground black pepper, to taste
1–2 sprigs fresh parsley for garnish (optional)

Whisk eggs and herbs in a small bowl. Stir in cooked seafood. Heat olive oil in a medium skillet over medium heat. Sauté garlic and vegetables for 1-2 minutes. Pour egg mixture into the skillet; scramble until cooked. Garnish with parsley (optional).

guac-o-money omelet

Serves 1
312 Calories; 3g CHO; 18g FAT; 26g PRO; 1g Fiber

- 2   cage free eggs
- 1   tablespoon milk or soymilk
- 1   teaspoon extra virgin olive oil
- ¼   cup turkey deli meat (nitrate free), chopped
- 2   tablespoons avocado, mashed
- 1   teaspoon lemon or lime juice

Note: *Feel free to substitute your favorite guacamole recipe for the mashed avocado and lemon or lime juice.*

Mix eggs and milk. Heat olive oil in a nonstick skillet. Pour in egg mixture. Sprinkle turkey meat on egg mixture in skillet. Scramble until cooked. Combine avocado and lemon or lime juice. Serve eggs with a spoonful of the avocado mixture on top.

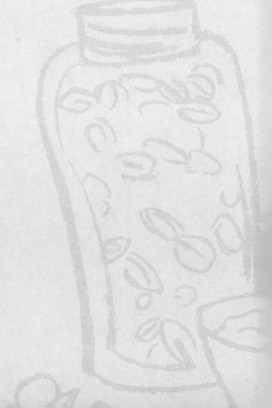

quiche

Serves 2
263 Calories per serving; 13g CHO; 15g FAT; 19g PRO; 3g Fiber

1	tablespoon extra virgin olive oil
4	egg whites (free-range)
2	whole eggs (free-range)
1	cup soy milk
½	cup sliced onion
½	cup chopped broccoli
½	cup sliced mushrooms
¼	teaspoon freshly-ground black pepper

Preheat oven to 325°. Coat quiche dish with oil. Mix egg whites and whole eggs with milk and pour into quiche dish. In a small skillet, sauté onion in a small amount of oil until it begins to brown; add broccoli and mushrooms. Continue to sauté until all the water from the mushrooms is gone and the vegetables are soft (about 4 minutes). Add pepper. Cool slightly and add to egg mixture in quiche dish. Stir to distribute evenly. Bake for 30 to 45 minutes or until knife inserted into center comes out clean.

broccoli quiche

2 large servings
246 Calories per serving; 22g CHO; 12g FAT; 12g PRO; 7g Fiber

1	redskin potato (small, 4-ounce), scrubbed, thinly sliced
1	tablespoon extra virgin olive oil
1	cup thinly-sliced shiitake, Portobello, and/or button mushrooms
2	medium onions, thinly sliced
1	garlic clove, minced
1	cup chopped broccoli
2	whole eggs plus 4 egg whites (free-range), beaten
	sea salt and freshly-ground black pepper to taste
¼	teaspoon dried basil
	salsa

Preheat oven to 325°. Steam potato in a large covered skillet for 4 minutes. Coat a 9-inch pie pan or quiche dish with 1 teaspoon olive oil, and distribute potato slices evenly across bottom. Heat remaining olive oil in small skillet over medium-high heat; sauté onion, mushrooms and garlic for 5 minutes, adding broccoli for last 2 minutes. Distribute this mixture over potato slices in quiche pan. In a small bowl, beat eggs with a fork. Add seasonings and pour over vegetables. Bake for 30 minutes or until center is set. Remove from oven and let rest for 5 minutes. Serve topped with salsa. (Quiche and frittata are great with a salad for lunch or a light dinner.)

asparagus quiche

Serves 2
300 Calories per serving; 24g CHO; 15g FAT; 18g PRO; 6g Fiber

1   redskin potato (small, 4 ounces), scrubbed, thinly sliced
1   tablespoon extra virgin olive oil
½   cup chopped onion
8   asparagus spears (8 ounces), cut into 2-inch pieces
1   cup chopped mushrooms,
3   eggs (free-range)
2   tablespoons grated Parmesan cheese (optional)
1   tablespoon chopped fresh chives,
½   teaspoon sea salt
⅛   teaspoon freshly-ground black pepper
     salsa

Preheat oven to 325°. Steam potato in large covered skillet for 4 minutes. Oil a 9-inch pie pan or quiche dish with 1 teaspoon olive oil, and distribute potato slices evenly across bottom. Heat remaining olive oil in small skillet over medium-high heat; sauté onion, asparagus, and mushrooms for 5 minutes. Distribute this mixture over potato in quiche pan. In a small bowl, beat eggs with a fork. Add seasonings and pour over vegetables. Bake for 30 minutes or until center is set. Remove from oven and let rest for 5 minutes. Serve topped with salsa

frittata

2 servings
290 Calories per serving; 18g CHO; 16 FAT; 20g PRO; 4g Fiber

1   tablespoon extra virgin olive oil
1   cup combined chopped green peppers, mushrooms, onions
1   garlic clove, minced
1   small unpeeled redskin potato, cut in ¼-inch pieces
8   asparagus spears, cut into 1-inch pieces
2   ounces cooked, uncured, nitrate-free turkey ham, ¼-inch dice
2   whole eggs plus 4 egg whites (free-range)
¼   cup (1 ounce) shredded part-skim mozzarella or reduced-fat sharp cheddar or
    Parmesan cheese
    sea salt and freshly-ground black pepper, to taste
    *(For additional servings, add 1 egg plus 2 egg whites per serving and increase other
    ingredients accordingly.)*

Heat oil in a 10-inch, oven-safe sauté pan over medium heat. Add vegetables
and meat and sauté for 15 seconds. Add 2-3 tablespoons water. Cover and steam
until vegetables are cooked through (about 2-3 minutes). Uncover, keep cooking,
stirring occasionally, until liquid evaporates and ingredients start to brown.
Combine and whisk together eggs, cheese, salt and pepper. Pour egg mixture over
vegetable mixture. Finish cooking using one of these two methods:

• Cover and cook over low heat for 7 minutes or until almost set, lifting edges
  and tilting sauté pan as eggs cook to allow uncooked portion to flow underneath.
  Then broil 5½ inches from heat for 1 minute or until eggs are set. Let stand for
  5 minutes.

• Cook over low heat without stirring for 1 minute. Transfer sauté pan to 325°
  oven and bake until frittata is puffed and set, about 10-12 minutes. Let stand for
  5 minutes.

Variation: Replace vegetable mixture with
1   cup broccoli florets
½   cup sliced yellow or zucchini squash
⅓   cup corn
2   ounces cooked, uncured, nitrate-free turkey ham, chopped

whole grain pancakes

Makes 6 pancakes
I pancake = 93 Calories; 14g CHO; 3g FAT; 4g PRO; 2g Fiber

I   egg (free-range), slightly beaten
⅔   cup water
½   tablespoon almond oil
I   cup *Whole Grain Baking Mix* (p 52)
½   teaspoon cinnamon
½   cup fresh or frozen blueberries

In a medium bowl, combine egg, water and oil. Add *Baking Mix* and beat with whisk until well blended. Brush a griddle, electric fry pan or large skillet with almond oil and preheat over medium heat (375°). Pour about 1/4 cup batter onto griddle for each pancake. Sprinkle with some blueberries. Cook for 2-3 minutes or until light brown on underside, then turn over and cook until second side is light brown.

oatmeal pancakes

10 pancakes, Serves 3-4
I pancake = 98 Calories; 15g CHO; 2g FAT; 5g PRO; 2g Fiber (excluding fruit topping)

2   tablespoons soy milk
5   egg whites (free-range)
2   whole eggs (free-range)
1½ cups rolled oats
½   cup low-fat cottage cheese
½   cup natural unsweetened applesauce
½   teaspoon vanilla extract
½   teaspoon cinnamon
½   tablespoon extra virgin olive oil

Mix all ingredients except oil in a blender until smooth (add more milk for creamier batter). Pour into large bowl; let stand for 5 minutes. Pour ⅓ cup batter per pancake onto hot, oiled griddle. Cook until bubbles form, then flip. Serve topped with a spoonful of fruit or natural applesauce.

power pancakes

10 pancakes, Serves 3-4
1 pancake = 126 Calories; 16g CHO; 2g FAT; 11g PRO; 2g Fiber

1   cup whole grain flour (unbleached, unbromated)
½   tablespoon aluminum-free baking powder
4   egg whites (free-range)
1   whole egg (free-range)
½   cup soy or rice protein powder
½   tablespoon brown sugar
½   teaspoon cinnamon
½   ripe banana, mashed
¾   cup soy milk
¾   cup blueberries
1   teaspoon extra virgin coconut oil, melted

Mix all ingredients except berries and oil. Beat just until blended; don't over beat. If mixture is too stiff, add more milk. Fold fruit into batter. Lightly oil a non-stick griddle. Pour 1/3 cup batter per pancake onto griddle and cook until bubbles form, then flip.

waffles and fruit

6 waffles, Serves 3
2 waffles = 226 Calories; 27g CHO; 20g FAT; 7g PRO; 4g Fiber

2 eggs (free-range)
1 cup + 2 tablespoons soy milk
3 tablespoons extra virgin coconut oil
2 teaspoons honey
1½ cups whole grain flour (unbleached, unbromated)
1 tablespoon aluminum-free baking powder
½ cup fruit, sliced

In medium bowl, combine eggs, milk, oil and honey. Beat well with a wire whisk or electric mixer. In a separate bowl, sift together flour and baking powder. Add dry ingredients to egg mixture and beat well. Add more milk, if necessary. Add fruit to batter. Cook in preheated waffle iron.

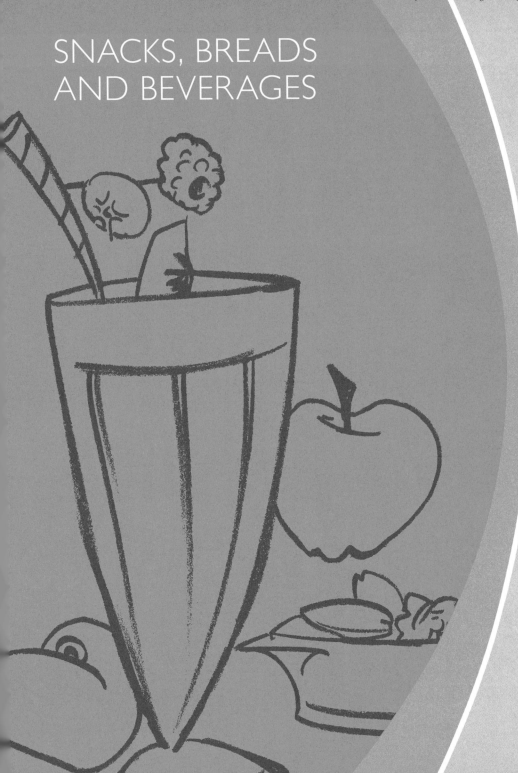

SNACKS, BREADS AND BEVERAGES

snacks, breads and beverages

 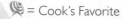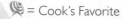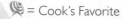
42

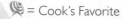 = Cook's Favorite

quick balanced snacks

175 to 250 calories per serving

- Low-fat cottage cheese + almonds, walnuts, flaxseed oil, or ground flaxseed
- Whole-grain bread + natural peanut butter, almond butter or extra virgin coconut oil
- Apple slices + natural peanut butter or almond butter
- Fruit serving + 5 almonds or walnuts
- Low-fat yogurt + flaxseed oil or ground flaxseed + fruit
- Tuna in water + canola mayonnaise + broccoli slaw + walnuts
- Rolled oats + raisins + almonds or walnuts (like trail mix)
- Fruit smoothie + flaxseed oil or extra virgin coconut oil + protein powder
- Whole grain rice cakes and extra virgin coconut oil
- Whole grain cracker + extra virgin coconut oil + fruit spread

trail mix

Serves 1
256 Calories per serving; 38g CHO; 8g FAT; 8g PRO; 6g fiber

⅓   cup rolled oats
1   tablespoon slivered almonds
⅛   cup raisins
     dash of cinnamon

Mix all ingredients and eat as a snack. To save time, make multiple servings; store in air-tight container.

energized bars

12 bars
1 bar = 200 Calories; 33g CHO; 4g FAT; 8g PRO; 3g Fiber

1   20-ounce can crushed pineapple in own juice
½   cup crushed almonds
2   cups rolled oats
3   scoops soy, rice or whey protein powder
1   cup chopped dried fruit
1½   teaspoons cinnamon

Preheat oven to 200°. Combine all ingredients. Spread in 13x9-inch pan brushed with expeller pressed canola oil. Bake for 90 minutes. Cool and slice. Store in refrigerator. Great snack anytime.

granola bars

20 bars
1 bar = 170 Calories; 23g CHO; 5g FAT; 8g PRO; 5g Fiber

2   very ripe bananas, mashed
2   tablespoons extra virgin coconut oil, melted
½   cup skim milk
1   cup natural unsweetened applesauce
3   tablespoons Stevia Plus™ blend
2   tablespoons honey
4   egg whites (free-range)
⅓   cup natural peanut butter
2   teaspoons vanilla extract
1   cup whole wheat flour (unbleached, unbromated)
⅓   cup ground flaxseed
2   teaspoons cinnamon
½   teaspoon ground nutmeg
½   teaspoon aluminum-free baking powder
¼   teaspoon sea salt
½   cup soy, rice or whey protein powder
1½ cups rolled oats
⅔   cup sprouted grain cereal (i.e. Ezekiel 4:9 Original®)
2   cups Uncle Sam™ cereal
1   cup dried fruit

Preheat oven to 350°. Brush a 9x13-inch glass pan with some coconut oil. In large bowl, combine bananas, oil, milk, applesauce, Stevia Plus™, honey, egg whites, peanut butter, and vanilla; mix well. Add flour, flaxseed, cinnamon, nutmeg, baking powder, salt, and protein powder; mix well. Stir in oats, cereals and dried fruit. Press mixture evenly into bottom of pan. For chewy bars, bake at 350° for 25 minutes, until the edges begin to brown. (For crunchy bars, bake at 300° until the surface is golden brown, about 45-50 minutes.) Remove from the oven and cool for 10 minutes. Cut into 20 bars. Allow to cool completely. Refrigerate or freeze (put bars in sandwich bags or plastic wrap, then in zip top freezer bags). Keeps nicely in freezer for up to 3 months. Thaw overnight in the refrigerator. Spread with 1 teaspoon natural peanut butter and serve with a glass of milk.

basic whole grain muffins

Serves 4
1 muffin = 206 Calories; 26g CHO; 8g FAT; 6g PRO; 4g Fiber

1   cup *Whole Grain Baking Mix* (p 52)
1   teaspoon aluminum-free baking powder
1   teaspoon cinnamon
1   egg white (free-range), slightly beaten
¼   cup skim milk
2   tablespoons extra virgin coconut oil, melted
2   tablespoons honey
½   teaspoon vanilla extract
½   cup fresh or frozen blueberries

Preheat oven to 400°. In a medium bowl, combine **Baking Mix,** baking powder, and cinnamon. In a small bowl, beat the egg white slightly; add the milk, oil, honey, vanilla and fruit. Pour the egg white mixture over the dry ingredients. Mix just until moistened. **Do not over stir** or muffins will be tough. Coat muffin tin with coconut oil. Spoon equal amounts of batter into each of 4 muffin cups. Bake about 18 minutes or until light brown. **Be careful not to over bake**, as this will dry out the muffins.

Variations: Replace the blueberries with one of these:

- ¼ cup raisins, ½ cup mashed banana, ¼ teaspoon nutmeg

- ¼ cup raisins, ⅔ cup chopped apple

- ½ cup chopped fresh pineapple with juice

peach oat bran muffins

Serves 12
1 muffin = 150 Calories; 19g CHO; 6g FAT; 5g PRO, 4g Fiber

1½   cups oat bran
½   cup whole grain flour (unbleached, unbromated)
2   teaspoons aluminum-free baking powder
1   teaspoon cinnamon
¼   teaspoon ground nutmeg
½   cup soy milk
⅓   cup honey
2   tablespoons almond oil
2   egg whites (free-range)
¼   cup slivered almonds
1   cup chopped fresh fruit

Preheat oven to 425°. Combine dry ingredients in a medium bowl and set aside.
In separate bowl, blend liquid ingredients. Pour liquid ingredients over dry
ingredients and mix just until blended. Do not over stir. Stir in almonds and fruit.
Coat muffin tin with oil. Pour equal amounts of batter into each of 12 muffin
cups. Bake for 18-20 minutes. Allow to cool slightly; remove from muffin tin to
cool completely.

🌸 flax bran muffins

Serves 12
1 muffin = 233 Calories; 34g CHO; 8g FAT; 8g PRO; 6g Fiber

1½   cups white whole wheat flour (unbleached, unbromated)
¾   cup ground flaxseeds
¾   cup oat bran
¼   cup brown sugar + 3 tablespoons Stevia Plus™
2   teaspoons baking soda
1   teaspoon aluminum-free baking powder
½   teaspoon sea salt
2   teaspoons cinnamon
1½   cups shredded carrots
2   apples, unpeeled, shredded
½   cup raisins
¾   cup chopped walnuts
3   egg whites (free-range)
¾   cup soy milk
1   teaspoon vanilla extract

Preheat oven to 350°. Combine flour, flaxseeds, oat bran, sugar, baking soda, baking powder, salt and cinnamon in a large bowl and mix well. Add carrots, apples, raisins and nuts. In a separate bowl, blend egg whites, milk and vanilla. Add liquid ingredients to dry ingredients; mix until just combined. Do not over stir. Coat muffin tin with coconut oil. Divide mixture into 12 muffin cups. Bake for 27-30 minutes. Allow to cool slightly; remove from muffin tin to finish cooling.

pita garlic bread

Serves 4
½ pita = 84 Calories; 15g CHO; 4g FAT; 2g PRO; 1g Fiber

2   whole grain pita bread
1   tablespoon extra virgin olive oil
2   garlic cloves, cut in half
¼   teaspoon dried oregano
1   tablespoon grated Parmesan cheese
    paprika
    sea salt

Cut each pita in half horizontally and lay on a cookie sheet or broiler pan. Brush each half with olive oil and rub with cut garlic. Sprinkle with oregano, Parmesan, paprika and sea salt. Broil for 1-2 minutes. Watch closely so it does not burn.

great cornbread

Serves 8
163 Calories per serving; 27g CHO; 4g FAT; 5g PRO; 4g Fiber

1½ cups yellow cornmeal
2   teaspoons aluminum-free baking powder
¼   teaspoon baking soda
½   teaspoon sea salt
¾   teaspoon Stevia Plus™ blend
1   tablespoon honey
1½ cups fat-free plain yogurt
2   tablespoons extra virgin coconut oil
2   egg whites (free-range)

Preheat oven to 425°. Brush a 9-inch round cake pan with expeller pressed canola oil. (Or heat a 9-inch cast iron skillet on the stovetop for 2 minutes on medium high heat; add 2 teaspoons expeller pressed canola oil, and proceed with recipe.) In a medium bowl, mix all the ingredients together just until well blended (do not beat or whip). Pour into cake pan or iron skillet; bake for 20-25 minutes. Allow to cool slightly. Cut into 8 wedges. Serve with organic butter. Great with bean soups or chili!

whole grain biscuits

Serves 3
1 biscuit = 178 Calories; 21g CHO; 8g FAT; 5g PRO; 3g Fiber

¾   cup *Whole Grain Baking Mix* (p 52)
½   teaspoon baking soda
2   teaspoons aluminum-free baking powder
2   tablespoons butter
⅓   cup skim milk (scant)

Preheat oven to 450°. Add *Baking Mix,* baking soda and baking powder to a medium bowl; cut butter into mix with 2 knives or pastry cutter, so mix is pea size. Add milk. Stir just until dough clings together. Drop 3 spoonfuls on an ungreased baking sheet. Bake about 10-11 minutes until light brown. These are NOT your grandma's biscuits! They are heavier, nuttier and much healthier.

whole grain bread crumbs

Makes 1 cup
270 Calories per serving; 57g CHO; 2g FAT; 12g PRO; 9g Fiber

Tear up 4 end crusts of sprouted whole grain bread; put 1-2 slices at a time in the blender. Pulse until the crumbs are consistently small. Pour into bowl and let sit on the counter for a few hours to dry. Put in a zip top bag and freeze for later use in *Gazpacho, Chicken Parmesan, Chicken Tenders, No-Fry Chicken, Oven Fried Chicken, Chicken Cordon Bleu, Fish Fingers, Crispy Cod,* or *Salmon or Tuna Patties* (see Index for page numbers).

whole grain baking mix

8 cups
1 cup = 405 Calories per serving; 79g CHO; 3g FAT; 17g PRO; 12g Fiber

- 2   cups sprouted grain cereal (Ezekiel 4:9 Original)
- 4   cups white whole wheat flour (unbleached, unbromated)
- 4   teaspoons vital wheat gluten
- 1   cup oat bran
- ½   cup organic, nonfat dry milk powder
- 2   tablespoons brown sugar
- 2   teaspoons Stevia Plus™ blend
- 3   tablespoons aluminum-free baking powder
- 1   teaspoon sea salt

Add cereal to food processor bowl with blade and pulse 6-10 times to break up the pieces. Add the remaining ingredients; pulse 6-10 times to blend. Store mix in a tightly covered container in the refrigerator to protect the flour from going rancid. Use in **Basic Whole Grain Muffins**, **Whole Grain Pancakes**, and **Whole Grain Biscuits** (see Index for page numbers).

sweet potato chips

Serves 2
97 Calories per serving; 13g CHO; 5g FAT; 1g PRO; 2g Fiber

- 1   medium sweet potato
      dash of sea salt
- 2   tablespoons extra virgin olive oil

Preheat oven to 450°. Cut potato into very thin (1/16-inch) slices. Place sliced potatoes in plastic bag with oil and salt. Shake well. Spread potatoes in a single layer on cookie sheet and bake for 7-10 minutes, turning 2-3 times. Remove chips as they brown.

turkey roll-up

3 roll-ups
1 roll-up = 140 Calories; 10g CHO; 8g FAT; 7g PRO; 1g Fiber

 3   slices deli turkey (nitrate-free)
15   almonds or walnuts, chopped
 1   small apple or kiwi, chopped

Spread turkey slices, layer remaining ingredients and roll-up.

CJ's smoothie

Serves 3 (16 ounces each)
194 Calories per serving; 24g CHO; 6g FAT; 11g PRO; 12g Fiber

 3   cups filtered water
 2   scoops soy, rice, hemp or whey protein powder
 1   16-ounce bag frozen unsweetened fruit
 1   banana
1½   tablespoons flaxseed oil or flaxmeal

Combine ingredients in blender. Cover and blend at high speed about 1 minute.
Keep refrigerated until served.

basic smoothie

Serves 1
195 Calories per serving; 19g CHO; 7g FAT; 18g PRO; 8g Fiber

⅔ cup filtered water*
1   cup unsweetened fresh or frozen** fruit
1   scoop natural flavor whey protein powder
1   tablespoon ground flaxseeds
¼ teaspoon cinnamon
¼ teaspoon vanilla extract
¼ teaspoon Stevia Plus™ blend (optional)

* If using fresh fruit, reduce water to ½ cup and add ⅓-½ cup crushed ice.

** If using frozen fruit, let it thaw slightly so it will move easily in the blender.

Put all the ingredients in a blender; process well, about 1 minute. Pour into large glass (share with others if you're a really nice person) and enjoy!

RK's piña colada smoothie

Serves 1
285 Calories per serving; 20g CHO; 15g FAT; 18g PRO; 1g Fiber

½ cup filtered water
1 cup fresh pineapple, cubed
1 scoop natural flavor soy, rice or whey protein powder
¼ teaspoon ground nutmeg
¼ teaspoon rum extract
¼ teaspoon Stevia Plus™ blend (optional)
½ cup crushed ice
1 tablespoon extra virgin coconut oil, melted

Add water, pineapple, protein powder, nutmeg, extract, Stevia Plus™ and ice to
the blender. Process for about 1 minute. Remove the cap in the blender cover,
restart the blender, and slowly pour the melted coconut oil into the smoothie. (This
prevents the oil from re-hardening in the smoothie.)

peach melba smoothie

Serves 1
190 Calories per serving; 18g CHO; 7g FAT; 18g PRO; 5g Fiber

⅔ cup filtered water
½ cup frozen peaches, partially thawed
½ cup frozen red raspberries, partially thawed
1 scoop natural flavor soy, rice or whey protein powder
¼ teaspoon ground cinnamon
¼ teaspoon vanilla extract
¼ teaspoon Stevia Plus™ blend
½ tablespoon flaxseed oil

Put all the ingredients in a blender; process well, about 1 minute

strawberry dream smoothie

Serves 2
305 Calories per serving; 24g CHO; 13g FAT; 23g PRO; 5g Fiber

2   cups frozen strawberries
1   cup soy or skim milk
3   tablespoons strawberry preserves
2   scoops soy, rice or whey protein powder
1½ tablespoons flaxseed oil

Combine ingredients in blender. Cover and blend at high speed about 1 minute.
Keep refrigerated until served.

KJ's chocolate smoothie

Serves 2 (8 ounces each)
314 Calories per serving; 32g CHO; 10g FAT; 24g PRO; 1g Fiber

1   cup Soy Delicious™ Frozen Dessert (chocolate velvet flavor)
1   cup carob soy milk
2   scoops soy, rice or whey protein powder
2   tablespoons whole almonds

Combine ingredients in blender. Cover and blend at high speed about 1 minute.
Pour into frosted glasses. Yum!

natural peanut butter smoothie

Serves 3 (8 ounces each)
240 Calories per serving; 15g CHO; 12g FAT; 18g PRO; 1g Fiber

1   cup orange juice
1   cup soy milk
2   tablespoons natural crunchy peanut butter
2   tablespoons flaxseed oil
2   scoops soy, rice or whey protein powder
½   teaspoon vanilla extract
1   cup ice

Combine ingredients in blender. Cover and blend at high speed until rich and creamy. Keep refrigerated until served.

berry blast smoothie

Serves 3 (12 ounces each)
249 Calories per serving; 17g CHO; 13g FAT; 16g PRO; 5g Fiber

2   cups filtered water
2   scoops soy, rice or whey protein powder
½   cup low-fat plain yogurt
2   tablespoons almond butter
1   cup frozen blueberries
1   cup frozen strawberries

Combine ingredients in blender. Cover and blend until rich and creamy.

Quick Tip: For a quick, easy cleaning of your blender after pouring out the smoothie, add 2 cups of warm-hot water and a few drops of dishwashing liquid to the blender; blend with cover on for 15 seconds. Dismantle the blender in the sink; rinse off the soap, drain, and your blender is clean and ready for next use.

applesauce plus

Serves 1
266 Calories per serving; 45g CHO; 6g FAT; 8g PRO; 6g Fiber

⅔   cup natural unsweetened applesauce
1   tablespoon dried fruit
1   tablespoon walnuts
1   tablespoon soy, rice or whey protein powder

Combine ingredients in a bowl and stir. Great anytime snack to satisfy that sweet
tooth. Balanced, easy and great tasting.

citrus mineral water

Serves 1

1   cup naturally carbonated or non-carbonated mineral water
1   teaspoon fresh-squeezed lemon or lime juice. slice of lemon or lime,
    or a splash of your favorite whole fruit juice

Pour over ice and enjoy.

cranberry mineral spritzer

Serves 1
15 calories; 4g CHO; 0g FAT, 0g PRO; 0g Fiber

1   cup naturally carbonated or non-carbonated mineral water
¼   cup natural, unsweetened cranberry juice

Pour over ice and enjoy.

pomegranate mineral spritzer

Serves 2
38 calories; 10g CHO; 0g FAT, 0g PRO; 0g Fiber

2   cups naturally carbonated or non-carbonated mineral water
¼   cup pomegranate juice

Pour over ice and enjoy.

berry good lemonade

Serves 2
35 Calories per serving; 11g CHO; 0g FAT; 1g PRO; 4g Fiber

2   cups filtered water, still or carbonated mineral water, chilled
1   cup fresh or frozen, cleaned red raspberries
5   tablespoons fresh lemon juice (2 medium lemons)
1½ teaspoons Stevia Plus™
4   large fresh mint leaves

Add all ingredients to blender; cover and blend on low speed for 15 seconds, then on high speed for 1 minute. Pour over ice cubes in glasses and garnish with additional mint leaves, if desired. (Make old-fashioned lemonade by omitting the berries and mint.)

hot cocoa

Serves 2
105 Calories per serving; 14g CHO; 1g FAT; 9g PRO; 0 Fiber

2   tablespoons unsweetened cocoa powder
2   teaspoons Stevia Plus™ blend
2   cups skim milk
    dash of cinnamon
    dash of sea salt
¼   teaspoon vanilla extract

In a small saucepan, combine the cocoa, Stevia Plus™, ½ cup milk, cinnamon, salt, and vanilla. Heat over medium heat, stirring constantly until mixture comes to a boil. Add remaining milk; heat through. Remove from heat and pour in mugs.

SALADS, DRESSINGS, DIPS, SAUCES AND SEASONINGS

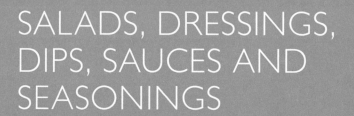

salads, dressings, dips, sauces and seasonings

 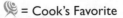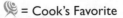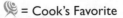
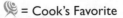 = Cook's Favorite

salad bar in a bag

Nutritional values vary depending on selection and quantity of ingredients and type of dressing used.

A great way to have a quick and healthy lunch, dinner or snack. Take a few minutes each week to wash and prepare your favorites from the following list and put each in its individual quart or gallon zip top bag. Line the bags up in the refrigerator. Also include any leftover roasted or grilled vegetables or meats. Have any frozen or canned items on hand.

When you are ready for a salad, grab your bowl, toss in a couple handfuls of greens, add a cup or more of vegetables and/or fruits, 2-3 ounces of protein, and a few nuts or seeds. Top with your favorite dressing, and you're good to go. Towards the end of the week, use up any leftover prepared vegetables in a stir-fry, roasted, or tossed in scrambled eggs, a quiche or frittata.

Greens	Vegetables	Fruits	Protein	Nuts/Seeds
Arugula	Alfalfa sprouts	Apple	Chicken, cubed	Almonds
Bibb lettuce	Artichoke hearts	Avocado	(poached, roasted,	Brazil nuts
Mesclun	Asparagus	Blueberries	pan-seared, grilled)	Ground flaxseeds
Romaine	Barley sprouts	Cherries, dried	Turkey, cubed	Peanuts
Spinach	Bean sprouts	Grapes	Salmon (poached,	Pine nuts
Swiss chard	Beans, green	Mandarin orange	roasted, grilled)	Pumpkin seeds
Watercress	Beets, sliced	Mango	Tuna, canned	Sunflower seeds
	Broccoli florets or slaw	Orange	Egg, boiled, chopped	Walnuts
	Cabbage (red or green)	Pear	Firm tofu, cubed	
	Carrots, sliced	Raisins	Low-Fat Cheeses:	
	Cauliflower florets	Strawberries	cheddar, swiss,	
	Celery, sliced		mozzarella, cottage	
	Cucumber, sliced		cheese, feta,	
	Mushrooms, sliced		Parmesan	
	Onions (red, green		Beans: black, red,	
	or white)		cannellini, garbanzo,	
	Parsnips		kidney	
	Peas, green			
	Peppers (red, green,			
	or yellow)			
	Radishes			
	Snow peas			
	Tomatoes			
	Water chestnuts			
	Leftover roasted or			
	grilled vegetables			

quinoa salad

2½ cups
½ cup = 211 Calories; 20g CHO; 13g FAT; 4g PRO; 3g Fiber

- 1   teaspoon lemon juice
- ¼   cup extra virgin olive oil
- 2   teaspoons fresh minced cilantro
- ½   teaspoon sea salt
- 1   cup fresh or frozen corn
- ¼   cup quinoa, rinsed thoroughly (brown rice, couscous, or bulgur may be substituted)
- ¼   teaspoon cumin
- ½   cup canned black beans, rinsed and drained
- 1   medium tomato, diced
- 1   tablespoon minced red onion

Make dressing by mixing lemon juice, oil, cilantro and salt in small, non-metal bowl; set aside. In a medium saucepan, cook the corn in 1 cup of water for 5 minutes. Remove the cooked corn to a bowl, reserving the liquid; set aside. Return corn-cooking liquid to a boil; add quinoa and cumin; cover and simmer until quinoa absorbs the liquid and is tender, about 10 minutes. Transfer quinoa to a large non-metal bowl; cool slightly. Add corn, remaining ingredients and dressing; toss. Chill and serve.

🌱 black bean mango salad

6 cups
1 cup = 214 Calories; 32g CHO; 6g FAT; 8g PRO; 10g Fiber

2	15-ounce cans black beans, rinsed and drained
1½	cups fresh or frozen corn, cooked
½	green bell pepper, chopped
½	red bell pepper, chopped
4	green onions, sliced thin
1	avocado, cubed
1	mango, cubed
2	tablespoons extra virgin olive oil
2	tablespoons balsamic vinegar

Mix all ingredients together. Refrigerate for 1 hour. One of my favorites.

65

zesty three bean salad

8 cups
3/4 cup = 173 Calories; 24g CHO; 5g FAT; 8g PRO; 6g Fiber

1	15-ounce can black beans
1	15-ounce can navy beans
1	15-ounce can red beans
2	medium limes, halved
1	12-ounce jar (1½ cups) medium salsa
2	tablespoons extra virgin olive oil
1	tablespoons chili powder
2	stalks celery, sliced
1	medium sweet onion, chopped or diced
1	medium tomato, diced

Prepare salad at least 30 minutes before serving. Drain and rinse beans and set aside. In a large bowl, squeeze lime juice; stir in salsa, oil and chili powder; mix well. Add drained beans, celery, onion and tomato; mix. Serve at room temperature. Store in refrigerator.

Stretched recipe: Use 3 large limes, 2 tablespoons chili powder, 1 full jar of salsa, 5 or 6 diced Roma tomatoes and 5 or 6 stalks of celery; substitute 1 large red onion for medium sweet onion. For spicier flavor, add hot pepper sauce to taste or cayenne pepper, sparingly.

taco salad

Serves 2
302 Calories per serving; 27g CHO; 13g FAT; 23g PRO; 10g Fiber (not including dressing)

1   cup *Basic Meat Sauce* (p 132)
1   tablespoon *Taco Seasoning* (p 79)
½   cup canned kidney beans, drained
3   cups Romaine, torn in pieces
1   small onion, sliced
1   small tomato, chopped
½   avocado, sliced
¼   cup shredded reduced-fat sharp cheddar
2   tablespoons low-fat sour cream
    tortilla chips made with expeller pressed canola oil
    or high-oleic safflower oil (optional)
    Taco Salad Dressing (p 76)

Combine *Basic Meat Sauce*, beans and *Taco Seasoning* in saucepan. Simmer uncovered for 10-15 minutes, stirring frequently. Arrange Romaine in 2 serving bowls. Top with simmered meat sauce, onion, tomato and avocado. Divide *Taco Salad Dressing* equally over 2 salads. Divide and add toppings of cheese and sour cream. Sprinkle with tortilla chips, if desired.

Variation: Omit the *Basic Meat Sauce*. Instead, use *Taco Seasoning* to make *Pan-Seared Chicken* (p 140) or *Pan-Seared Salmon* (p 171). Slice cooked chicken or break salmon into chunks. Top the Romaine with chicken or salmon, beans, onion, tomato and avocado. Proceed as above with remaining ingredients, beginning with dressing.

chicken salad

Serves 4
276 Calories per serving; 12g CHO; 12g FAT; 27g PRO; 3g Fiber

- 2 cups cooked chicken or turkey breast
  (grilled, poached, steamed or pan-seared), cubed
- 1 cup sliced green or red grapes
- ½ cup sliced green onion
- ½ cup sliced almonds
- 2 tablespoons canola mayonnaise

Combine all ingredients and chill. Serve over Romaine lettuce.

cherry chicken salad

Serves 4
264 Calories per serving; 12g CHO; 12g FAT; 27g PRO; 3g Fiber

- 1 pound boneless, skinless, chicken breast (grilled, poached, steamed or pan-seared), cut into 1-inch cubes
- ½ cup dried cherries
- ¼ cup canola mayonnaise blended with ½ teaspoon prepared mustard
- ¼ cup broken walnuts
- ¾ cup diagonally-sliced celery
- ⅛ cup chopped onion

Mix all ingredients. Serve on a bed of greens or fill a whole grain tortilla for a wrap sandwich.

chicken waldorf salad

Serves 1
337 Calories per serving; 26g CHO; 15g FAT; 27g PRO; 4g Fiber

3 ounces (¾ cup) cooked chicken breast, cubed
1 apple, cored and chopped
¼ cup chopped celery
1 tablespoon chopped onion
sea salt and freshly-ground black pepper, to taste

Dressing (whisk together):
1 tablespoon canola mayonnaise
½ tablespoon extra virgin coconut oil, melted

Toss ingredients together and eat. Best if eaten as soon as it's put together, otherwise coconut oil hardens.

chicken caesar salad

Serves 4
Salad = 180 Calories per serving; 7g CHO; 5g FAT; 29g PRO; 3g Fiber
3 T. Dressing = 65 Calories; 1g CHO; 5g FAT; 2g PRO; 0g Fiber

Marinade:
3   tablespoons fresh lemon juice
2   garlic cloves, minced

1   pound boneless, skinless chicken breast
8   cups Romaine lettuce, torn
2   large tomatoes, cut in eighths
½   cup sliced red onion, separated into rings
2   tablespoons grated Parmesan cheese
    Caesar Salad Dressing (p 75)

Mix marinade ingredients in zip top bag. Add chicken, seal bag and turn to coat chicken. Refrigerate for 30 minutes. Preheat outdoor grill or broiler. Prepare *Caesar Salad Dressing* in small bowl; whisk to blend well and set aside. Drain chicken and discard marinade. Grill or broil chicken for 5-6 minutes on each side, until juices run clear. In a large bowl, combine lettuce, tomatoes and onion. Pour dressing over salad; toss to coat. Slice chicken breasts and arrange on salad. Sprinkle with 2 tablespoons Parmesan cheese.

🌿 CJ's big salad

Serves I
367 Calories per serving; 24g CHO; 19g FAT; 25g PRO; 8g Fiber

I	tablespoons balsamic vinegar
I	tablespoon extra virgin olive oil
½	cup broccoli slaw
5	grape tomatoes
2	cups spinach or Romaine lettuce, torn
⅛	cup sliced red pepper
I	tablespoon raisins or dried cherries
½	tablespoon slivered almonds
I	6-ounce can tuna or wild salmon in water

Mix vinegar and oil together; set aside. Mix all other ingredients in a large bowl. Drizzle vinegar and oil mixture over top of salad; toss. This is my lunch two or three times per week; fast, easy, healthy and I love the taste.

salmon salad

Serves 4
346 Calories per serving; 18g CHO; 18g FAT; 28g PRO; 3g Fiber

8 tablespoons extra virgin olive oil, divided
4 tablespoons balsamic vinegar
　sea salt and freshly-ground black pepper to taste
¼ cup vegetable, chicken or fish broth
4 4-ounce salmon fillets
6 cups spinach or Romaine lettuce
2 tablespoons capers, drained
½ small red onion, thinly sliced
4 tablespoons cooked corn kernels

In a small bowl, whisk together 6 tablespoons oil and 3 tablespoons vinegar. Season with salt and pepper and set aside to use as dressing. Pour remaining oil and vinegar into a large sauté pan; add broth. Heat to a boil, reduce temperature and add salmon. Cover pan, poach for 10-15 minutes, and then transfer to a plate to cool. Prepare each serving plate with 1½ cups of greens. Add salmon fillet and garnish with capers, red onion and corn. Drizzle balsamic vinaigrette over each serving.

citrus salad

Serves 4-6
147 Calories per serving; 16g CHO; 7g FAT; 5g PRO; 5g Fiber

1	head red lettuce, torn
1	head Bibb or buttercrunch lettuce, torn
½	cup chopped celery
2	cans (2 cups) mandarin oranges, drained
½	cup chopped almonds
⅓	cup chopped green onion
½	cup chopped watercress sprigs
¼	cup chopped Italian flat leaf parsley
	Citrus Salad Dressing (p 75)

Mix all ingredients together and toss with *Citrus Salad Dressing.*

Variation: Substitute grapefruit sections or diced or sliced avocado for oranges

shrimp avocado salad

Serves 4
189 Calories per serving; 9g CHO; 10g FAT; 25g PRO; 5g Fiber (not including dressing)

1	pound peeled and deveined shrimp, cooked and chilled
6	cups assorted mixed greens
1	large avocado, peeled and sliced
1	large orange, peeled and sectioned
	So Simple Salad Dressing (p 74)

Arrange mixed greens in bowl. Top with avocado, orange and shrimp and drizzle with dressing.

so simple salad dressing

Serves 16
2 tablespoons = 116 Calories; 2g CHO; 12g FAT; 0g PRO; 0g Fiber

1   cup extra virgin olive oil
1   cup balsamic vinegar (or vinegar of choice)

Mix with a wire whisk. Store at room temperature. Always ready to serve.

apple flax vinaigrette

Serves 12
3 tablespoons = 126 Calorie; 1g CHO; 14g FAT; 0g PRO; 0g Fiber

¼   cup apple cider vinegar
2   teaspoons Dijon mustard
½   teaspoons ground coriander
½   teaspoon freshly-ground black pepper
½   cup flaxseed oil
¼   cup extra virgin olive oil
1   cup apple cider
2   tablespoons shoyu, tamari or reduced-sodium soy sauce
    or Bragg Liquid Aminos™

In a medium bowl, combine vinegar, mustard, coriander and pepper. Add oils and whisk together until well blended and emulsified. Whisk in cider and shoyu until well combined. Store in airtight container in the refrigerator for up to one week.

caesar salad dressing

12 tablespoons
3 tablespoons Dressing = 65 Calories; 1g CHO; 5g FAT; 2g PRO; 0g Fiber

⅓ cup low-fat sour cream
¼ cup canola mayonnaise
1 tablespoon grated Parmesan cheese
2 tablespoons chopped Italian flat leaf parsley
1 tablespoon skim milk
½ teaspoon freshly-ground black pepper
½ teaspoon Worcestershire sauce
1 tablespoon lemon juice
2 garlic cloves, minced
¼ teaspoon anchovy paste

Mix ingredients in a small bowl and whisk to blend well. Set aside until ready to dress salad.

citrus salad dressing

Serves 6
2 tablespoons = 166 Calories; 1g CHO; 18g FAT; 0g PRO; 0g Fiber

½ cup extra virgin olive oil
⅛ cup tarragon vinegar
⅛ cup lemon juice
½ teaspoon Worcestershire sauce
1 teaspoon sea salt
  freshly-ground black pepper, to taste
  dash of hot pepper sauce (optional)

Blend thoroughly with a wire whisk.

greek salad dressing

Serves 16
2 tablespoons = 134 Calories; 2g CHO; 14g FAT; 0g PRO; 0g Fiber

- ¾ cup extra virgin olive oil
- ¾ cup expeller pressed canola oil
- ⅔ cup garlic-flavored red wine vinegar
- 2 tablespoons honey
- 2 teaspoons sea salt-based seasoned salt
- 1 teaspoon dried sweet basil
- 1 teaspoon dry mustard
- 1 teaspoon freshly-ground black pepper

Mix all ingredients in a blender or food processor. Refrigerate. (Extra virgin olive oil will get harder and somewhat cloudy in the refrigerator, so let mixture sit at room temperature or run the container under warm water for a few minutes before using.) This is also a great meat marinade.

taco salad dressing

Serves 2
90 Calories per serving; 3g CHO; 7g FAT; 2g PRO; 1g Fiber

- 1 tablespoon extra virgin olive oil
- 2 tablespoons red wine vinegar
- ¾ cup mild salsa

Whisk ingredients together in a small bowl. Pour equal amounts over two salads.

red pepper dip

2 cups
I tablespoon = 37 Calories; 5g CHO; Ig FAT; 2g PRO; < .5g Fiber

2   medium red bell peppers, halved lengthwise
I   large red onion, cut in 1/4-inch slices
2   garlic cloves, peeled
¼   cup dry **Whole Grain Bread Crumbs** (p 51)
¼   cup plain low-fat yogurt
I   tablespoon red wine vinegar
2   teaspoons extra virgin olive oil
¼   cup chopped fresh cilantro (optional)

Place pepper halves, skin sides up, on a foil-lined cookie sheet. Arrange onion slices and garlic around peppers. Broil 6-8 inches from heat source until vegetables are blackened, about 10 minutes. Place vegetables in paper bag; seal and let stand for 15 minutes. Remove vegetables from bag. Remove blackened skin of peppers. In food processor, combine peppers, onion and garlic; process until finely chopped. Add remaining ingredients and process until smooth. Transfer mixture to bowl. Fold in cilantro, season with salt and pepper to taste and serve. Store in refrigerator.

bean dip

5 cups
1/2 cup = 160 Calories; 28g CHO; 4g FAT; 3g PRO; 6g Fiber

I   recipe of **Refried Beans** (p 179) (or I 30-ounce can of fat-free refried beans)
I   4-ounce can diced green chilies
I   cup salsa

Mix ingredients together in large skillet or saucepan and heat through. Delicious on a whole wheat tortilla for a burrito or used in **Nachos** (p 149) or **Taco Salad** (p 67). Freezes well.

tartar sauce 1

8 tablespoons
1 tablespoon = 66 Calories; < 1g CHO; 7g FAT; 0g PRO; <.1g Fiber

2   tablespoons extra virgin coconut oil, melted
¼   cup canola mayonnaise
2   tablespoons minced onion

Whisk ingredients together thoroughly in a small bowl just before serving with fish. Leave at room temperature. Best if used fresh, as the coconut oil hardens when refrigerated.

tartar sauce 2

5 tablespoons
1 tablespoon = 58 Calories; 1g CHO; 6g FAT; 0g PRO; < .1g Fiber

¼   cup canola mayonnaise
1   dill pickle, chopped

Mix together in small bowl; serve.

horseradish sauce

Serves 2
3 tablespoons = 40 Calories; 2g CHO; 2g FAT; 2g PRO; 0g Fiber

4   tablespoons low-fat sour cream
1   tablespoon horseradish
1   tablespoon chopped fresh chives

Whisk ingredients together thoroughly in a small bowl just before serving. Very good with grilled venison or buffalo.

herbes de provence

8 teaspoons
4 Calories per serving; < Ig CHO; <.Ig FAT; < .Ig PRO; < .2g Fiber

4   teaspoons dried thyme
2   teaspoons dried marjoram
1   teaspoon dried rosemary
2   teaspoons dried savory
1   bay leaf

Put in blender or Mini-Mate Cuisinart and pulse 10 -15 times. Store in airtight container. Can be used in homemade *Dry Onion Soup Mix* (p 110).

taco seasoning

33 Calories per serving; < .Ig FAT; < .I g PRO; < .I g Fiber
Makes 2 tablespoons, equivalent to using I packet of purchased taco seasoning

2   teaspoons instant minced onion
1   teaspoon sea salt
1   teaspoon chili powder
½   teaspoon arrowroot
¼   teaspoon dried red pepper, crushed
½   teaspoon garlic powder
¼   teaspoon dried oregano
½   teaspoon ground cumin

Put in blender or Mini-Mate Cuisinart and pulse 10 times. Store in an airtight container. Use for tacos, *Southwestern Soup, Taco Salad, Refried Beans, Pan-Seared Chicken, Chicken Fajitas*, or *Nachos* (see Index for page numbers).

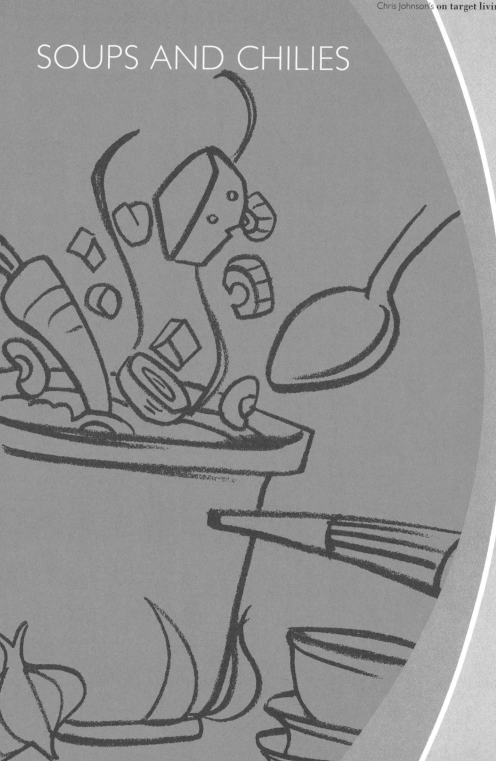

SOUPS AND CHILIES

soups and chilies

🍲 = Cook's Favorite

refried bean soup

5 cups
I cup = 130 Calories; 21g CHO; 3g FAT; 7g PRO; 5g Fiber

- 2 teaspoons extra virgin olive oil
- I garlic clove, minced
- ½ cup chopped onion
- I 14.5-ounce can Italian stewed tomatoes
- I 15-ounce can fat-free refried beans
- 1½ cups chicken broth

In large skillet, heat olive oil over medium-high heat; sauté garlic and onion in olive oil for 5 minutes. Add remaining ingredients and heat through. To serve, sprinkle with additional chopped onion, tomato, and avocado.

tortilla soup

6 cups
1 cup = 184 Calories; 26g CHO; 5g FAT; 8g PRO; 5g Fiber

1	tablespoon extra virgin olive oil
1	large onion, chopped
1	jalapeño pepper, seeded and finely chopped
1	garlic clove, minced
1	small zucchini, sliced ½-inch thick
1	cup canned whole tomatoes, drained and chopped
3	cups low-sodium vegetable broth
1	15-ounce can black beans, rinsed and drained
½	teaspoon dried oregano
2	tablespoons fresh lime juice
4	tablespoons shredded cheese
4	teaspoons chopped fresh cilantro (optional)
2	cups yellow tortilla chips made with high oleic safflower oil

In large saucepan, heat oil over medium-high heat. Add onion, jalapeño and garlic and cook, stirring often, until onion is slightly soft, about 4-5 minutes. Add zucchini, tomatoes, broth, black beans and oregano. Cook, stirring occasionally, until zucchini is almost soft, about 3 minutes. Stir in lime juice. Ladle soup into bowls and top each serving with cheese, cilantro and tortilla chips. Serve hot.

two-bean soup

9 cups
I cup = II3 Calories; 2Ig CHO; Ig FAT; 6g PRO; 6g Fiber

2 teaspoons extra virgin olive oil
I large onion, chopped
I medium green pepper, chopped
4 cloves garlic, minced
I 15-ounce can kidney or black beans, drained
I 15-ounce can fat-free refried beans
2 cups chicken broth
I 14.5-ounce can Italian stewed tomatoes
¾ cup salsa
2 teaspoons chili powder
½ teaspoon pepper
¼ teaspoon ground cumin

In large skillet, heat olive oil over medium-high heat; sauté onion, green pepper, and garlic for 5 minutes. Add remaining ingredients and heat through.

autumn soup

8 cups
1 cup = 139 Calories; 17g CHO; 3g FAT; 14g PRO; 4g Fiber

1½ cups beef broth
¼ cup pearled barley
½ tablespoon extra virgin olive oil
1 cup chopped onion
½ cup sliced carrots
¼ cup sliced celery
2 garlic cloves, chopped
2 cups *Basic Meat Sauce* (p 132)
2 cups beef broth
½ cup chopped mushrooms
½ cup chopped cabbage
¼ cup green beans
½ cup unpeeled redskin potatoes, cut in ½-inch cubes
½ tablespoon steak sauce
¼ teaspoon dried thyme
   sea salt and freshly-ground black pepper, to taste
1 14.5-ounce can Italian stewed tomatoes

In a large saucepan, simmer pearled barley in 1½ cups beef broth covered for 45 minutes. Meanwhile, in large skillet, heat oil over medium-high heat; sauté onions, carrots, celery, and garlic for 5-10 minutes. At the end of the 45 minutes, add the sautéed vegetables and *Basic Meat Sauce* to the cooked barley. Add the remaining 2 cups beef broth, mushrooms, cabbage, beans, potatoes, steak sauce, thyme, salt and pepper; simmer covered for 20 minutes. Add the tomatoes and heat through.

fast chili

6 cups
1 cup = 177 Calories; 25g CHO; 3g FAT; 14g PRO; 7g Fiber

1   tablespoon extra virgin olive oil
1   cup chopped onion
1   14.5-ounce can Italian stewed tomatoes
2   cups *Basic Meat Sauce* (p 132)
1   15-ounce can kidney, black, or pinto beans, rinsed and drained
½   tablespoon chili powder (more to taste)

In a large skillet, heat olive oil over medium-high heat; sauté onion for 5 minutes.
Add remaining ingredients, bring to boil, cover and simmer for 10-15 minutes.

slower chili

6 cups
1 cup = 173 Calories; 20g CHO; 4g FAT; 15g PRO; 6g Fiber

½   tablespoon extra virgin olive oil
10   ounces ground buffalo
1   cup chopped onion
1   cup chopped green pepper
2   teaspoons minced garlic
1   15-ounce can kidney, black, or pinto beans, rinsed and drained
1   14.5-ounce can stewed tomatoes
1   8-ounce can tomato sauce
1   cup beef broth
½   cup filtered water
½   cup frozen corn (optional)
½   tablespoon chili powder
½   teaspoon cumin
½   teaspoon dried oregano
1   teaspoon dried cilantro
    sea salt and freshly-ground black pepper, to taste

In a large skillet, heat olive oil over medium-high heat and brown meat. Add onions, green pepper and garlic and brown another 5 minutes. Transfer mixture to a large soup pot and add remaining ingredients. Simmer 30 minutes. Sprinkle with chopped avocado, onion, tomato, and/or cheese to serve. Best if made a day ahead. This freezes very well for up to 3 months.

minestrone soup

10 cups
1 cup = 161 Calories; 17g CHO; 4g FAT; 13g PRO; 4g Fiber

1   tablespoon extra virgin olive oil
1   pound ground buffalo
1   cup diced onion
2   garlic cloves, minced
½   cup sliced carrots
2   14.5-ounce cans Italian stewed tomatoes
3   cups beef broth
1   cup finely-shredded cabbage
1   15-ounce can cannellini, black or great northern beans, rinsed and drained
1   teaspoon dried oregano
½   teaspoon dried thyme
½   teaspoon sea salt
     freshly-ground black pepper
1   small zucchini, cut in 1/4-inch slices
1   ounce whole grain capellini
1   teaspoon dried sweet basil
     Parmesan cheese (optional)

In a large skillet, heat olive oil over medium-high heat and brown meat. Add
onions, garlic and carrots and brown another 5 minutes. Transfer mixture
to a large soup pot; add tomatoes, beef broth, cabbage, beans and seasonings.
Simmer 30 minutes. Add zucchini, pasta and basil; simmer for 10 minutes.
Sprinkle with Parmesan cheese to serve (optional).

✿ southwestern bean soup

8 cups
1 cup = 155 Calories; 23g CHO; 3g FAT; 11g PRO; 4g Fiber

1   tablespoon extra virgin olive oil
2   cups chopped onion
2   cups **Basic Meat Sauce** (p 132)
1   cup frozen corn
1   15-ounce can black or red beans, rinsed and drained
1   14.5-ounce can Italian stewed tomatoes
1   tablespoon **Taco Seasoning** (p 79)
½   cup water or broth

In a large skillet, heat olive oil over medium-high heat and sauté onions for 5 minutes. Add **Basic Meat Sauce** and remaining ingredients; simmer for 20-30 minutes.

basic meat for stew

½ recipe (3 cups meat + 1½ cups liquid)
½ recipe = 1,005 Calories per serving; 10g CHO; 39g FAT; 156g PRO; 0 fiber

 3 pounds boneless buffalo shoulder, trimmed of fat,
    cut into 1½ to 2-inch chunks
 2 tablespoon extra virgin olive oil
1½ cups chopped onion
 1 tablespoon garlic, minced
 4 cups beef broth
 ½ teaspoon sea salt
    freshly-ground black pepper

Heat oil in large fry pan over medium-high heat. Add meat cubes and brown
in 1-pound batches. Return all the meat to the pan. Add onions and garlic and
sauté for 5 minutes. Add broth, salt and pepper, scraping pan to release browned
bits. Bring to boil; cover. Reduce heat and simmer for 2 to 2½ hours until meat
is tender. Divide meat and liquid into two equal portions. Proceed with recipe for
Classic Stew (p 92) or *Tex-Mex Meat Stew* (p 93), or store portions for later use.
Can be refrigerated for up to 3 days; frozen in airtight containers for up to
3 months.

SOUPS AND CHILIES

91

classic stew

8 cups
1 cup = 192 Calories; 14g CHO; 5g Fat; 23g PRO; 4g fiber

1	teaspoon extra virgin olive oil
12	ounces crimini or button mushrooms (4 cups), cleaned, trimmed and cut in half
1	large onion, cut in 8 pieces
10	small redskin potatoes (2 cups), scrubbed and quartered
1	pound carrots (3 cups), peeled, cut in 1½-inch chunks
⅛	head small cabbage (2 cups), chopped
1	cup beef broth
¾	cup tomato juice
½	recipe of **Basic Meat for Stew** (p 91) (about 3 cups meat and 1½ cups liquid)
½	teaspoon dried thyme
1	tablespoon dried parsley
1	teaspoon ground dry mustard
	sea salt and freshly-ground black pepper to taste
1	tablespoon whole wheat flour (unbleached, unbromated)

Heat oil in large fry pan over medium-high heat and sauté mushrooms for
5 minutes. Add all ingredients except flour. Bring to boil; cover, reduce heat
to low and simmer for 20-30 minutes until vegetables are tender. (Can also put
all ingredients in clay cooker and bake in oven for 75 minutes at 325°.) Mix flour
with 2 tablespoons of water; stir into hot stew. Continue cooking for 5 minutes
longer until thickened. Serve with *Whole Grain Biscuits* (p 51).

tex-mex meat stew

8 cups
1 cup = 220 Calories; 21g CHO; 6g FAT; 24g PRO; 5g fiber

½ recipe of **Basic Meat for Stew** (p 91) (about 3 cups meat and 1½ cups liquid)
2 cups fresh or frozen corn
1 15-ounce can black beans, rinsed and drained
1 4-ounce can chopped green chilies
½ teaspoon garlic powder
½ teaspoon chili powder
½ teaspoon oregano
1 8-ounce can tomato sauce
1 tablespoon whole wheat flour (unbleached, unbromated)

Put **Basic Meat for Stew**, corn, beans, chilies and seasonings into a large saucepan. Bring to a boil over medium-high heat. Whisk flour into tomato sauce. Stir into stew and simmer uncovered for 5 minutes, until stew thickens. Serve with **Great Cornbread** (p 50).

SOUPS AND CHILIES

93

chicken stew

Serves 4
406 Calories per serving; 30g CHO; 18g FAT; 31g PRO; 4g Fiber

1	tablespoon extra virgin olive oil
1	garlic clove, pressed
1	large onion, chopped
1	pound boneless, skinless chicken breast, cut into 2-inch cubes
4	large carrots, sliced
6	small redskin potatoes, cut in ½-inch cubes
1	15-ounce can tomatoes, chopped
1	teaspoon cinnamon
	pinch of cayenne pepper
1	teaspoon ground cumin
2	tablespoons natural chunky peanut butter
1½	cups chicken broth
	sea salt and freshly-ground black pepper, to taste

In large skillet, sauté garlic and onion in olive oil. Add chicken and brown. Add remaining ingredients, except chicken broth, and stir until blended. Add broth and seasonings to taste. Bring to a boil. Cover, reduce heat and simmer until sauce thickens, about 50 minutes.

cream of mushroom soup with chicken

5 cups
1 cup = 234 Calories; 21g CHO; 10g FAT; 16g PRO; 2g Fiber

- 1 tablespoon extra virgin olive oil
- 1 pound fresh mushrooms, sliced
- ½ cup chopped onion
- 2 cups lower-sodium chicken broth
- 1 cup fat-free evaporated milk, divided
- 1½ tablespoons arrowroot
- 12 ounces raw (or 8 ounces cooked) boneless, skinless chicken breast, cut into ½-inch cubes
  freshly-ground black pepper
- 1 tablespoon chopped fresh Italian flat leaf parsley or 1 teaspoon dried

If chicken is not already cooked, heat ½ tablespoon olive oil in a large skillet over medium heat and brown chicken about 2 minutes; remove from skillet and set aside. Add ½ tablespoon olive oil to the skillet; sauté mushrooms and onion until tender. Transfer half of these vegetables to a blender, add broth and process until smooth. Return mixture to the skillet. In small bowl, stir arrowroot and ¼ cup milk until smooth; add to the skillet. Add remaining ¾ cup milk and cubed chicken to the skillet. Cook and stir over medium heat until soup thickens. Sprinkle with parsley and serve.

Variation: pour over thinly-sliced, unpeeled redskin potatoes and onions to make scalloped potatoes; bake about 1 hour at 350°.

nancy's mexican soup

9 cups
1 cup = 163 Calories; 24g CHO; 3g FAT; 13g PRO; 6g Fiber

8 ounces boneless, skinless chicken breast
3 cups chicken broth
1 cup chopped onion
2 garlic cloves, minced
1 tablespoon extra virgin olive oil
1 15-ounce can fat-free refried beans
1 15-ounce can black beans, rinsed and drained
1½ cups frozen corn, thawed
1¼ cups salsa
   chili powder to taste
   freshly-ground black pepper

Bring broth to boil in saucepan. Drop in chicken, cover and simmer on low heat for 10-15 minutes. Remove chicken from the pan to cool and set broth aside to cool, as well. Cut cooled chicken into cubes. In a small skillet, heat olive oil over medium-high heat; sauté onion and garlic for 5 minutes. Add chicken cubes, sautéed onion and garlic to the broth in the saucepan. Add remaining ingredients and heat through for 10 minutes to cook the corn.

white chicken chili

10 cups
1 cup = 128 Calories; 11g CHO; 4g FAT; 12g PRO; 3g Fiber

1   tablespoon extra virgin olive oil
1   large onion, chopped
1   red or green pepper, chopped
2   garlic cloves, minced
1   15-ounce can white beans, rinsed and drained
3   cups chicken broth, divided
2   cups cooked chicken breast, cubed
1   14.5-ounce can Italian stewed tomatoes
2   teaspoons chili powder
1   teaspoon cumin
1   teaspoon dried oregano
    sea salt and freshly-ground black pepper, to taste
1   ounce (¼ cup) reduced-fat cheese, shredded (optional)

In large skillet, heat olive oil over medium-high heat and sauté onion, pepper, and garlic for 3-5 minutes. Meanwhile, put 1 cup of beans and 1½ cups chicken broth in blender, and blend until smooth. Add all the beans, chicken, remaining broth and seasonings to skillet. Simmer for 15 minutes. Serve in bowls, each sprinkled with 1 tablespoon reduced-fat shredded cheese. (Best if made ahead and allowed to steep; freezes well.)

quick chicken chili

Serves 6-8
292 Calories; 17g CHO; 12g FAT; 29g PRO; 4g Fiber

1 pound cooked boneless, skinless chicken breast, cubed
1 15-ounce jar great northern beans, rinsed and drained
1 12-ounce jar salsa
   sea salt and freshly-ground black pepper to taste

Combine all ingredients in a large saucepan. Heat thoroughly. Fast and easy.

fast chicken noodle soup

10 cups
1 cup = 121 Calories; 9g CHO; 5g FAT; 12g PRO; 2g Fiber

1	tablespoon extra virgin olive oil
1	cup cdiced elery
1	cup chopped onion
1½	cups chopped carrots
2	garlic cloves, minced
8	cups chicken broth
½	teaspoon sea salt
	freshly-ground black pepper
½	teaspoon dried thyme, crushed
¼	teaspoon dried oregano, crushed
½	teaspoon poultry seasoning
1	pound boneless, skinless chicken breast
1	cup (2 ounces) fine whole wheat noodles
1	cup frozen green peas

In large skillet, heat olive oil over medium-high heat; sauté celery, onion, carrots, and garlic for 5 minutes. Add broth, salt, pepper, thyme, oregano, poultry seasoning and chicken. Bring to boil; reduce heat, cover and simmer for 5 minutes. Uncover and return broth to a boil. Add noodles and peas and bring to a boil again. Reduce heat, cover and simmer for 12 minutes. Remove chicken from broth and cut into cubes; return chicken to broth; heat through. Ready to serve. (Freezes well.)

SOUPS AND CHILIES

99

ostrich soup

Serves 6
336 Calories per serving; 25g CHO; 12g FAT; 32g PRO; 5g Fiber

  2   teaspoons extra virgin olive oil
1½   pounds ground ostrich
  1   onion, chopped
  1   green bell pepper, chopped
  ½   red bell pepper, chopped
  4   garlic cloves, minced
 32   ounces tomato puree
 32   ounces filtered water
  2   cups sliced green beans
  2   cups chopped kale or spinach
  1   cup chopped celery
      sea salt and freshly-ground black pepper, to taste

Heat oil in a soup pot over medium heat. Add meat and brown, stirring to separate meat particles and incorporate brown bits. Add onion, bell peppers and garlic; cook until tender (about 5 minutes). Add remaining ingredients and simmer for 20 minutes. This is an excellent tasting, nutritious soup. Give it a try.

sweet potato minestrone

10.5 cups
I cup = 184 Calories; 23g CHO; 5g FAT; 11g PRO; 5g Fiber

2	teaspoons extra virgin olive oil
½	pound lean ground turkey
1	cup sliced onion
1	cup diced carrots
¾	cup thinly-sliced celery
3	cups chicken broth
2	cups peeled, diced sweet potato
2	14.5-ounce cans no-salt-added whole tomatoes, chopped, undrained
1	15-ounce can great northern beans, rinsed and drained
1	teaspoon dried oregano
½	teaspoon freshly-ground black pepper
¼	teaspoon sea salt
8	cups coarsely-chopped spinach

Heat olive oil in a large saucepan over medium-high heat. Add meat, onion, carrots and celery, and sauté for 7 minutes, stirring to separate meat particles and incorporate brown bits, or until meat is browned. Add broth and all remaining ingredients, except spinach. Bring to a boil; cover, reduce heat and simmer for 15 minutes or until vegetables are tender. Stir in spinach; cook an additional 2 minutes.

turkey chili

16 cups
1 cup = 160 Calories; 10g CHO; 8g FAT; 13g PRO; 7g Fiber

1 tablespoon extra virgin olive oil
1 pound ground turkey breast
2 onions, diced
1 teaspoon garlic, minced
1 cup shredded carrots
1 red pepper, chopped
1 green pepper, chopped
2 15-ounce cans garbanzo beans, rinsed and drained
1 15-ounce can kidney beans, rinsed and drained
½ teaspoon red pepper flakes
½ teaspoon cayenne pepper
1 tablespoon chili powder
1 teaspoon dried oregano
1 tablespoon ground cumin
2 32-ounce bottles low-sodium vegetable blend juice
1 14.5-ounce can stewed tomatoes

Heat oil in a large pot over medium-high heat. Add turkey, onions, garlic, carrots, peppers; sauté for 5 minutes, stirring to separate meat particles. Add remaining ingredients; bring to a boil and cover. Reduce heat to low and simmer for 15 minutes.

See *Potato Soup with Turkey Ham and Peas* under *Basic Potato Soup variations* (p 106).

SOUPS AND CHILIES

salmon asparagus chowder

6 cups
1 cup = 252 Calories; 19g CHO; 9g FAT; 24g PRO; 4g Fiber

2 cups chicken broth
3 cups asparagus spears, washed/trimmed, cut into 1½-inch pieces
1 recipe **Pan-Seared Salmon** (p 170)
1 tablespoon extra virgin olive oil
1 large leek (or 2 bunches of green onions)
1 cup chopped carrots
1 cup chopped celery
1 cup cubed, unpeeled redskin potatoes
2 garlic cloves, minced
1 bay leaf
½ teaspoon thyme
   sea salt and freshly-ground black pepper, to taste
2 cups skim milk
4 tablespoons shredded reduced-fat sharp cheddar
2 tablespoons finely minced fresh chives

In large skillet, bring chicken broth to a boil, add asparagus to and cook about 5 minutes. Drain and reserve broth. Plunge asparagus into ice water to prevent overcooking; then drain. Strain broth and set aside. In same skillet, heat olive oil over medium-high heat. Add leeks or onions and sauté 4 minutes. Add celery, garlic, and carrots and sauté 1 minute more. Add potatoes, strained broth, bay leaf, thyme, salt and pepper. Simmer uncovered until potatoes are quite tender, about 15 minutes. Let cool slightly and then mash at least half of the vegetables in the pot. Add milk and heat just to a boil. Add reserved asparagus and chunks of salmon. Stir very gently so salmon remains in chunks. Continue to cook for 5 additional minutes over low heat. Ladle into bowls and garnish with reduced-fat cheddar cheese and chives.

cod and green pea chowder

5 cups
1 cup = 256 Calories; 23g CHO; 7g FAT; 20g PRO; 4g Fiber

Follow instructions for *Salmon Asparagus Chowder*, replacing the salmon with 12 ounces of cooked cod and the asparagus with 1 cup of fresh or frozen green peas.

clam chowder

9 cups
1 cup =153 Calories; 19g CHO; 5g FAT; 9g PRO; 1g Fiber

Make *Basic Potato Soup* (p 105). After mashing half of the potatoes, add 2 cans chopped clams, drained, along with the remaining ingredients. Cover and heat through, but do not boil.

basic potato soup

8 cups
I cup = 148 Calories; 21g CHO; 5g FAT; 5g PRO;2g Fiber

2   tablespoons extra virgin olive oil
I   cup chopped onion
½   cup chopped or julienned carrots
½   cup chopped celery
½   cup chopped cabbage
4   cups raw, unpeeled redskin potatoes, cut in ½-inch cubes
2   cups chicken broth
2   cups skim milk
½   teaspoon dried sweet basil
½   teaspoon sea salt
    freshly-ground black pepper
I   tablespoon butter
I   tablespoon dried parsley flakes

In large skillet, heat olive oil over medium-high heat; sauté onion, carrots, celery and cabbage for 10 minutes. Add potatoes and broth. Cover and simmer 15-20 minutes, until potatoes are soft, stirring occasionally to prevent potatoes sticking to bottom of skillet. Mash half of the potatoes while still in the skillet. Add remaining ingredients, cover and heat through, but do not boil. Very best if it seasons overnight; freezes well. Can be served with garnish of 1 tablespoon reduced-fat cheese.

Variations: This is a very versatile soup. Add any of your favorite protein (tuna, cooked salmon, cooked chicken, etc.) and vegetables (fresh spinach, kale, broccoli, etc.). Some variations include *Clam Chowder* (p 104), *Asparagus Chowder, Corn Chowder* and *Potato Soup with Turkey Ham and Peas* (recipes on p 106).

asparagus chowder

10 cups
1 cup = 127 Calories; 19g CHO; 4g FAT; 5g PRO; 2g Fiber

Make *Basic Potato Soup* (p 105). After mashing half of the potatoes, add 2 cups cooked fresh or frozen asparagus along with the remaining ingredients. Cover and heat through, but do not boil.

🌹 corn chowder

10 cups
1 cup = 154 Calories; 25g CHO; 5g FAT; 5g PRO; 2g Fiber

Make *Basic Potato Soup* (p 105). After mashing half of the potatoes, add 2 cups cooked fresh or frozen corn along with the remaining ingredients. Cover and heat through, but do not boil.

potato soup with turkey ham and peas

10 cups
1 cup = 140 Calories; 21g CHO; 4g FAT; 7g PRO; 3g Fiber

Make *Basic Potato Soup* (p 105). After mashing half of the potatoes, add 4 ounces cubed turkey ham steak (uncured, no nitrates, 96 precent fat free) and 1½ cups cooked fresh or frozen peas along with the remaining ingredients. Cover and heat through, but do not boil.

gazpacho

Serves 4
196 Calories; 26g CHO; 8g FAT; 5g PRO; 6g Fiber

1	small can tomato paste
2	cans water
2	small garlic cloves
1	green pepper, coarsely chopped
1	red pepper, coarsely chopped
1	yellow pepper, coarsely chopped
1	medium onion, coarsely chopped
2	fresh tomatoes, diced, or 1 14.5-ounce can diced tomatoes, drained
2	tablespoons red wine vinegar
1	large cucumber, coarsely chopped
½	cup **Whole Grain Bread Crumbs** (p 51)
2	tablespoons extra virgin olive oil

Put tomato paste and water into blender or food processor and blend until mixed. Add remaining ingredients. Use "chop" button until everything is well mixed. Pour soup into a bowl. Add bread crumbs and stir until well blended. Chill and serve.

SOUPS AND CHILIES

107

gazpacho, too

6 cups
1 cup = 74 Calories; 12g CHO; 3g FAT; 3g PRO; 3g Fiber

4   cups tomatoes, unpeeled, cored, seeded, quartered
2   cups chopped cucumber
1   cup chopped onion
1   cup chopped green pepper
2   tablespoon red wine vinegar
1   tablespoon extra virgin olive oil
1   heaping tablespoon chopped fresh sweet basil
½   teaspoon sea salt
¼   teaspoon freshly-ground black pepper
2   garlic cloves, minced
1   cup water
    ice cubes

Combine everything except water and ice cubes in a food processor; pulse 8-10 times or to desired consistency. (If using a blender, combine the ingredients in a large bowl and blend 2 cups at a time in the blender to desired consistency, pouring blended portions into a second bowl.) Pour mixture into a medium bowl; stir in water. Cover and chill at least 1 hour. Serve with an ice cube floating in each serving bowl.

garden vegetable soup

6 cups
1 cup = 74 Calories per serving; 11g CHO; 3g FAT; 3g PRO; 3g Fiber

1	tablespoon extra virgin olive oil
1	cup sliced carrots
½	cup chopped onion
1	stalk celery, chopped
2	garlic cloves, minced
1½	cups sliced fresh mushrooms
2	cups chicken or beef broth
¾	cup diced green cabbage
½	cup green beans
1	14.5-ounce can Italian stewed tomatoes
1	tablespoon lemon juice
½	tablespoon steak sauce
½	teaspoon dried basil
¼	teaspoon dried oregano
¼	teaspoon dried thyme
¼	teaspoon sea salt
	freshly-ground black pepper

In a large skillet, heat olive oil over medium-high heat; sauté carrots, onion, celery, garlic, and mushrooms for 10 minutes. Add remaining ingredients and simmer covered 15 minutes. (Can also add ½ cup spinach, Swiss chard ribbons, kale, Brussels sprouts, cauliflower, broccoli, rinsed/drained sauerkraut, etc.)

Quick Tip: One teaspoon of dried herbs is equal to 1 tablespoon of fresh herbs; use whichever is available.

cream soup mix

equivalent to 1 can of condensed soup
185 Calories per serving; 34g CHO; < 1g FAT; 12g PRO; 1g Fiber

To use in place of canned cream soups in casseroles or as a base for other soups. Much lower in fat and salt than the canned versions.

¼ cup powdered nonfat milk
2 tablespoons arrowroot
½ tablespoon instant sodium-free chicken bouillon
1 tablespoon dried onion flakes
¼ teaspoon dried basil
¼ teaspoon dried thyme
   freshly-ground black pepper

Combine all ingredients, mixing well. To substitute for one can of condensed soup: Combine the dry mix with 1¾ cups cold water in saucepan. Cook and stir until thickened. Add to casserole as you would the canned product. Can be made in multiple batches and stored in an airtight container. If using from a multiple batch, measure out ⅓ cup mix and proceed as above.

dry onion soup mix

Makes 2 tablespoons - equivalent of 1 package of dry onion soup mix
108 Calories per serving; 21g CHO; 2g FAT;3 g PRO; 2g Fiber

4 teaspoons low-sodium beef or chicken bouillon granules
3 tablespoons dried, minced onion
1 teaspoon onion powder
½ teaspoon *Herbes de Provence* (p 79)

Mix together and store in airtight container. Mix with 1½ cups low-fat sour cream for vegetable dip. Sprinkle over roast or chicken before baking.

ENTRÉES

entrées

Chicken and Turkey

Fish and Seafood

🌸 = Cook's Favorite

basic sandwich

Serves 1
190 Calories per serving; 22g CHO; < 1g FAT; 4g PRO; 4g Fiber

2 slices whole grain bread
  Romaine lettuce leaves
  Tomato and onion slices
  Sandwich filling of your choice (add to above nutritional values)

tuna salad sandwich filling

Serves 1
170 Calories per serving; 0 g CHO; 9g FAT; 21g PRO; < 1g Fiber

3 ounces tuna, drained
1 tablespoon canola mayonnaise
½ teaspoon mustard
2 tablespoons chopped onion

Mix ingredients together. Spread on bread; add vegetables; slice and eat.

egg salad sandwich filling

Serves 1
162 Calories per serving; 1g CHO; 12 FAT; 10g PRO; < 1g Fiber

1 whole boiled egg + 1 boiled egg white (free range), chopped
1 tablespoon canola mayonnaise
½ teaspoon mustard

Mix ingredients together. Spread on bread; add vegetables; slice and eat.

chicken salad sandwich filling

Serves 1
227 Calories per serving; 0g CHO; 11g FAT; 27g PRO; < 1g Fiber

3 ounces cooked boneless, skinless chicken breast, chopped
1 tablespoon canola mayonnaise
½ teaspoon mustard
2 tablespoons chopped onion

Mix ingredients together. Spread on bread; add vegetables; slice and eat.

stuffed pita

Serves 4
½ pita = 202 Calories; 25g CHO; 11g FAT; 4g PRO; 6g Fiber

½ cup prepared hummus
4 cups *Basic Roasted Vegetables* (p 180)
2 whole grain pitas, cut to create half moons

Roast your preferred combination of vegetables per recipe or use leftover roasted vegetables. Spread each pita half with 2 tablespoons hummus and fill with ¼ of the vegetables.

ENTRÉES

115

sloppy joes

Serves 7-8
125 Calories per serving; 7g CHO; 5g FAT; 14g PRO; 1g Fiber (not including roll or bread)

2	tablespoons extra virgin olive oil
1	pound ground turkey
1	cup chopped onion
½	cup chopped celery
1	15-ounce can tomato sauce
2	tablespoons rolled oats
1	teaspoon Worcestershire sauce
½	teaspoon chili powder
	dash of hot pepper sauce
½	cup water
1	teaspoon sea salt
⅛	teaspoon freshly-ground black pepper
	whole grain rolls or bread (1 per serving)

In large skillet, heat oil over medium-high heat and sauté turkey, onion and celery until browned. Stir in tomato sauce, oats, Worcestershire sauce, chili powder, hot pepper sauce, water, salt and pepper. Simmer uncovered about 30 minutes. Spoon about ½ cup of mixture onto each roll or slice of bread.

sloppy joes, too

Serves 4
107 Calories per serving; 9g CHO, 2g FAT; 14g PRO; 2g Fiber (not including roll)

2 cups *Basic Meat Sauce* (p 132)
¼ cup chopped green bell pepper
¼ cup chopped onion
2 teaspoons brown sugar
2 teaspoons apple cider vinegar
1 teaspoon Worcestershire sauce

Combine all the ingredients in a medium saucepan and bring to a boil. Reduce heat and simmer uncovered for 20 minutes. Spoon onto a whole grain or sprouted grain roll.

vegetarian bbq

Serves 6
291 Calories per serving; 32g CHO; 3g FAT; 34g PRO; 3g Fiber (including the roll)

1 10.5-ounce package frozen bite-size soy meat substitute, thawed
1 garlic clove, minced
1 tablespoon tomato paste
1 medium onion, finely chopped
1 cup barbecue sauce
1 tablespoon brown mustard
1 teaspoon maple syrup
1 tablespoon extra virgin olive oil
6 whole grain rolls or hamburger buns

Chop soy meat substitute into ½-inch pieces. Place in bowl with all ingredients except olive oil and rolls. Set aside and let stand for 10 minutes so flavors meld. Grill whole grain rolls or buns for 2-4 minutes. In medium skillet, heat oil over medium-high heat and add soy meat mixture. Reduce heat and simmer, stirring occasionally, for about 10 minutes (until sauce thickens). Spoon mixture over rolls or buns and serve. Can be frozen in single servings.

ENTRÉES

117

chicken quesadillas

Serves 4
385 Calories per serving; 51g CHO; 9g FAT; 25g PRO; 4g Fiber

1 tablespoon extra virgin olive oil
¾ pound boneless, skinless chicken breast
1 large red or green pepper, chopped
1 medium onion, chopped
½ teaspoon *Taco Seasoning* (p 79)
2 large whole grain lavash (no hydrogenated oils)
1 cup mild salsa
½ cup low-fat cheddar cheese
1 large tomato, diced

Heat 1 teaspoon oil in a large skillet over medium heat. Cut chicken into small chunks; sauté until cooked through (about 3 minutes). Add peppers and onion and continue to sauté, about 3 more minutes. Sprinkle with *Taco Seasoning*, remove and set aside. Heat 1 teaspoon oil in skillet. Place 1 lavash in skillet. Scatter half the chicken, vegetables, cheese and salsa over one-half of the lavash. Fold other half of lavash over chicken mixture. Heat on medium until bottom is lightly browned. Turn over and heat until cheese melts. Remove from skillet. Repeat with second lavash. Cut into triangles.

confetti wrap

Serves 2
264 Calories per serving; 21g CHO; 9g FAT; 26g PRO; 3g Fiber

2   tablespoons canola mayonnaise
½   teaspoon mustard
1   6-ounce can boneless, water-packed, wild-caught skinless salmon, drained
1   package broccoli slaw mix
½   small onion, diced
2   whole grain tortillas (no hydrogenated fats)

Blend mayonnaise and mustard. Add remaining ingredients and mix well.
Enjoy as a salad or wrap in tortillas. For variety, add sliced grapes or a few
broken walnuts.

turkey burgers or meatloaf

Serves 8
199 Calories per serving; 13g CHO; 7g FAT; 21g PRO; 3g Fiber

1½ pounds lean ground turkey
1 10-ounce package frozen chopped spinach (thawed and drained)
2 eggs whites (free-range)
1½ teaspoons Italian seasoning
1 cup rolled oats
½ cup chopped onion
½ cup shredded carrots
1 small apple, shredded
⅓ cup skim milk
½ teaspoon sea salt
¼ teaspoon freshly-ground black pepper

Preheat oven to 350°. Combine all ingredients in a large bowl and mix thoroughly. Shape into loaf in 9x13-inch baking pan. Bake for 45-50 minutes or until internal temperature reaches 160°. Let stand 5 minutes before slicing.

For burgers, form into patties and broil, bake or grill as desired.

Optional: Spread ¼ cup tomato salsa on meatloaf during last 15 minutes of baking.

chicken and vegetable pizza

8 slices
1 slice = 230 Calories; 23g CHO; 8g FAT; 21g PRO; 4g Fiber

1   pound boneless, skinless chicken breast, cut in 1/2-inch cubes
1   tablespoon extra virgin olive oil
1   small onion, sliced
½   green bell pepper, sliced
½   red bell pepper, sliced
⅓   cup mango, pineapple, or peach chutney or salsa
1   8-ounce can pineapple tidbits, drained
1   cup (4 ounces) shredded reduced-fat mozzarella cheese
1   12-inch, ready-made, thin whole grain pizza crust

Preheat oven to 450°. Heat oil in large skillet; sauté chicken, onion and peppers until chicken is no longer pink. Spread chutney evenly on ready-made pizza crust. Spread chicken mixture and pineapple tidbits over chutney and sprinkle cheese on top. Bake for 10-12 minutes and cut into 8 slices.

ENTRÉES   121

mexican pizza

Serves 2
343 Calories per serving; 40g CHO; 13g FAT; 15g PRO; 9g Fiber

1   tablespoon extra virgin olive oil
2   8-inch whole grain tortillas (no hydrogenated oils)
½   cup salsa, drained
¼   cup canned red kidney beans, rinsed and drained
¼   cup canned black beans, rinsed and drained
1   tablespoon chopped fresh cilantro
⅓   cup shredded reduced-fat hot pepper Monterey Jack cheese

Preheat oven to 375°. Coat a cookie sheet lightly with olive oil. Place tortillas on the cookie sheet. Brush each tortilla with oil. Spoon half the salsa onto each tortilla and sprinkle with beans, cheese and cilantro. Bake 10-15 minutes or until cheese melts.

pita pizza

4 halves
½ pita = 310 Calories; 30g CHO; 11g FAT; 17g PRO; 5g Fiber

1	small zucchini, sliced diagonally
1	large onion, sliced
1	small red pepper, sliced
2	mushrooms, sliced
1	tablespoon extra virgin olive oil
	sea salt and freshly-ground black pepper, to taste
2	whole grain pitas, cut in half horizontally
1	cup pizza sauce
2	ounces uncured, nitrate-free turkey ham
4	ounces part-skim mozzarella cheese (1 cup shredded)

Preheat oven to 450°. Place prepared vegetables on lightly-oiled cookie sheet. Sprinkle with remaining olive oil, salt and pepper. Roast vegetables for 10-15 minutes, turning once. Remove from the oven. Reduce oven heat to 400°. Lay 4 pita halves on cookie sheet or perforated pizza pan; brush lightly with olive oil. Top each pita with ¼ of the sauce, ham, roasted vegetables, and cheese. Bake for 10 minutes. Remove from oven and let rest 2 minutes before serving.

Quick Tip: Use 3-4 cups of leftover *Roasted Vegetables* (p 180) instead of preparing these vegetables from scratch.

beef with bok choy

Serves 4
280 Calories per serving; 8g CHO; 16g FAT; 28g PRO; 3g Fiber

12 ounces beef sirloin, sliced in thin strips
2   tablespoons reduced-sodium soy sauce
1   tablespoon rice wine
½   teaspoon baking soda
2   teaspoons arrowroot
2   garlic cloves, minced
1   teaspoon toasted sesame oil
2   tablespoons extra virgin coconut oil, divided
4   cups bok choy, cut in 1-inch chunks
1   can sliced water chestnuts, drained
½   cup julienned carrots
¼   pound snow pea pods
1   onion, sliced
½   cup mushrooms, sliced
⅓   cup chicken broth
1   tablespoon arrowroot

In a medium bowl, combine meat, soy sauce, rice wine, baking soda, arrowroot, garlic and sesame oil; set aside for 15-20 minutes. In large skillet, heat 1½ teaspoons oil over medium-high heat and stir-fry bok choy for 2-3 minutes. Remove from skillet to a bowl. Heat 1½ teaspoons coconut oil and stir-fry water chestnuts, carrots, pea pods, onion and mushrooms for 2 minutes. Remove from skillet to bowl with bok choy. Heat remaining 1 tablespoon of coconut oil; stir-fry meat mixture for 2-3 minutes. Add the vegetables back into the skillet. In a small bowl, mix the chicken broth and 1 tablespoon arrowroot. Add to the skillet and heat through until the broth thickens.

beef and green bean stir-fry

Serves 3
345 Calories per serving; 7g CHO; 21g FAT; 31g PRO; 3g Fiber

1	2 pound green beans, trimmed and left whole
1	tablespoon extra virgin coconut oil
9	ounces beef sirloin, sliced in thin strips
½	tablespoon grated fresh gingerroot
1	garlic clove, minced
¼	cup beef broth
2	tablespoons natural peanut butter
1½	tablespoons red wine vinegar
1½	tablespoons reduced-sodium soy sauce
1	teaspoon toasted sesame oil
1	tablespoon chopped peanuts

In covered, medium saucepan, cook beans in 1 inch of water for 6 minutes. Plunge hot beans into cold water to stop cooking; drain and set aside. In large skillet, heat oil over medium-high heat and stir-fry meat, gingerroot, and garlic for 3-5 minutes. Whisk together broth, peanut butter, vinegar, soy sauce, and sesame oil; add to beef and cook until thickened. Add cooled beans and heat. Transfer mixture to serving bowl and sprinkle with chopped peanuts.

steak spinach stir-fry

Serves 2
360 Calories per serving; 28g CHO; 15g FAT; 32g PRO; 11g Fiber

6	ounces buffalo steak, sliced in thin strips
½	tablespoon paprika
1	tablespoon extra virgin coconut oil
1	garlic clove, minced
1	onion, chopped
¾	cup beef broth
½	pound (about 8 cups) spinach, washed, stemmed
½	cup sliced green onions with tops
½	cup sliced mushrooms
½	cup fresh bean sprouts
¼	cup water
1	tablespoon reduced-sodium soy sauce
2	tablespoons arrowroot
¼	teaspoon minced gingerroot

Sprinkle meat with paprika. In large skillet, heat coconut oil over medium-high heat and sauté meat. Add garlic and onion and sauté for 2 minutes. Add broth and remaining vegetables; sauté for 3 minutes. Stir together water, soy sauce, arrowroot and gingerroot. Add to meat and vegetables and stir until thickened.

ENTRÉES   125

steak kew with pea pods, broccoli or asparagus

Serves 2
386 Calories per serving; 29g CHO; 16g FAT; 31g PRO; 8g Fiber

- 6 ounces buffalo steak, sliced in thin strips
- 6 green onions, chopped
- 1 tablespoon reduced-sodium soy sauce
- 1½ tablespoons hoisin sauce
- 1 teaspoon toasted sesame oil
- 1 teaspoon arrowroot
- 1 teaspoon minced garlic
- ¼ teaspoon gingerroot, minced
  freshly-ground black pepper
- 1 tablespoon extra virgin coconut oil, divided
- 1 cup snow pea pods
- 1 carrot, julienned
- ½ pound mushrooms, sliced
- 1 cup fresh bean sprouts
- 1 can water chestnuts, drained

In a medium bowl, combine meat, onions, soy sauce, hoisin sauce, sesame oil, arrowroot, garlic, gingerroot, and pepper; let stand at least 15 minutes. In large skillet, heat half the coconut oil over medium-high heat; stir-fry pea pods, carrot, and mushrooms for 2 minutes. Add bean sprouts and water chestnuts to heat through. Remove from skillet to bowl. Heat remaining coconut oil in skillet. Stir-fry meat mixture for 1-2 minutes. Add vegetables and heat through.

szechuan beef and snow peas

Serves 2
306 Calories per serving; 13g CHO; 15g FAT; 29g PRO; 5g Fiber

6   ounces beef sirloin, sliced in thin strips
1   tablespoon arrowroot
3   tablespoons rice wine
2   tablespoons teriyaki sauce
½   teaspoon hot red pepper flakes
½   teaspoon toasted sesame oil
1   teaspoon minced gingerroot
1   garlic clove, minced
1   tablespoon extra virgin coconut oil, divided
2   cups snow pea pods
1   red pepper, sliced
2   stalks celery, sliced diagonally
6   green onions, cut into 1½-inch pieces

Combine meat, arrowroot, rice wine, teriyaki sauce, pepper flakes, sesame oil, gingerroot and garlic in medium bowl; let stand at least 15 minutes. In large skillet, heat half the oil over medium-high heat; stir-fry pea pods, pepper, celery, and onions for 2-3 minutes. Remove from skillet to a bowl. Heat remaining oil and stir-fry meat mixture for 3 minutes. Add vegetables and heat through.

ENTRÉES   127

marinated meat kebabs

Serves 8
200 Calories per serving; 7g CHO; 4g FAT; 36g PRO; 1g Fiber (excluding the marinade)

Marinade
½   cup extra virgin olive oil
¼   cup balsamic vinegar
¼   cup chopped onion
3   garlic cloves, minced
1   teaspoon sea salt
1   teaspoon freshly-ground black pepper
2   teaspoons lower sodium soy sauce

2   pounds venison steak, cut in 1½- to 2-inch cubes
16 whole mushrooms
2   onions cut in quarters
2   green peppers, cut in 1½- to 2-inch squares
2   zucchinis, cut in 1-inch chunks
8   small redskin potatoes, parboiled for 10 minutes
½   cup barbecue sauce

In a zip top plastic bag, combine marinade ingredients and mix well; add meat cubes. Seal the bag, expelling excess air, and squeeze the bag until all the cubes are coated with the marinade. Refrigerate a minimum of 3 hours to overnight, turning the bag occasionally. Prepare the vegetables. Drain the meat and discard the marinade. Using metal skewers, thread the meat cubes alternating with a variety of vegetables. (If using bamboo skewers, be sure to soak them in water for 20 minutes before making the kebabs to prevent burning.) Grill on medium-high heat for 2-3 minutes on each of 4 sides. Brush barbecue sauce on kebabs about 1 minute before removing from the grill.

pan-seared buffalo medallions

Serves 2
1 medallion without sauce = 235 Calories; 0g CHO; 13g FAT; 32g PRO; 0g Fiber

1	tablespoon extra virgin olive oil
2	5-ounce buffalo medallions, ¾-inch thick
	sea salt and freshly-ground black pepper, to taste

Heat olive oil in an 8-10-inch heavy skillet over medium heat. Sprinkle medallions with salt and pepper and place in skillet. Cook without moving the medallions until they are browned, approximately 3 minutes for well done (1½-2 minutes for rare). Using a metal spatula, turn medallions over and cook on the second side an additional 3 minutes for well done (1½-2 minutes for rare). Transfer medallions to warm plate, tent with foil so some air can circulate, and let rest for 5 minutes. To serve, spoon your sauce of choice over the top of each medallion.

Prepare one of the following sauces by mixing in a small bowl.

Lemon-Garlic Sauce

1	tablespoon butter (room temperature)
1	tablespoon fresh parsley, minced
½	teaspoon lemon zest, grated
1	small garlic clove, minced.

Horseradish Sauce

2	tablespoons low-fat sour cream
1	tablespoon horseradish

🥀 buffalo/turkey meatloaf

Serves 8
187 Calories per serving; 10g CHO; 6g FAT; 16g PRO; 4g Fiber

1   medium onion, finely chopped
1   medium carrot, finely chopped
4   medium mushrooms, finely chopped
1   garlic clove, minced
½   cup cooked beans or lentils, mashed
8   ounces ground turkey breast
8   ounces ground buffalo
¾   cup salsa, divided
1   egg (free-range)
¼   cup skim milk
¾   teaspoon Italian herb mix
¼   teaspoon sea salt
    freshly-ground black pepper
½   tablespoon regular mustard
½   tablespoon Worcestershire sauce
2   tablespoons extra virgin olive oil
¾   cup rolled oats

Preheat oven to 350°. Put meats in a medium bowl. Add chopped vegetables, mashed beans, ½ cup of salsa, and remaining ingredients. Mix thoroughly. Lightly coat a 9x4-inch bread pan with olive oil and shape meatloaf in pan. Bake for 35 minutes. Spread remaining ¼ cup salsa on top of meatloaf and continue baking 35 minutes more or until internal temperature is 160°. **Do not over bake.**

buffalo roast with vegetables

Serves 6
425 Calories per serving; 51g CHO; 8g FAT; 43g PRO; 10g Fiber

1	tablespoon extra virgin olive oil
1	boneless, rolled buffalo shoulder roast (2 pounds)
3	cups beef broth
4	tablespoons dried onion
1	garlic clove, minced
½	teaspoon **Herbes de Provence** (p 79)
	sea salt and freshly-ground black pepper to taste
6	medium redskin potatoes, scrubbed and halved
6	medium carrots, peeled and halved
6	medium onions, peeled
6	wedges of cabbage
1½	tablespoons arrowroot (optional)

Heat oven to 350°. Heat olive oil in large skillet over medium heat. Add roast to skillet, and brown both sides. Transfer the roast to a small roasting pan or covered clay pot. Mix broth, onion, garlic and seasonings in skillet. Pour over the roast. Cover and roast in oven for 2 hours. Add prepared vegetables. Cover and roast for an additional 1¼ hours. Broth may be thickened with arrowroot to make gravy.

ENTRÉES

131

🌹 basic meat sauce

8 cups
1 cup = 185 Calories; 12g CHO; 3g FAT; 28g PRO; 3g Fiber

1	tablespoon extra virgin olive oil
2	pounds ground buffalo
2	cups chopped onion
1	cup chopped celery
4	large garlic cloves, minced
2	14.5-ounce cans Italian stewed tomatoes
1	14.5-ounce can beef broth
1	6-ounce can tomato paste
1½	teaspoons hot sauce
½	teaspoon freshly-ground black pepper
½	teaspoon dried thyme
1	teaspoon dried sweet basil
⅛	teaspoon sea salt
2	bay leaves
¼	cup chopped fresh Italian flat leaf parsley

ENTRÉES

In a large skillet, brown meat (one pound at a time) in olive oil. Add onion, celery and garlic and sauté for 5 more minutes. Stir in tomatoes, broth, tomato paste, hot sauce, pepper, thyme, basil, salt, and bay leaves. Bring to a boil; reduce heat, and simmer uncovered for 35 minutes, stirring occasionally. Stir in parsley; cook another 2 minutes. Discard bay leaves. This is a very versatile recipe—use in *Sloppy Joes, Too*; *Fast Chili, Spanish Rice, Sauce for Spaghetti or Lasagna, Goulash, Southwestern Bean Soup, Autumn Soup, Taco Salad*; (see Index for page numbers). Can be frozen in 2-cup portions in zip top bags for up to 3 months.

sauce for spaghetti or lasagna

6 cups
1 cup = 182 Calories; 22g CHO; 5g FAT; 14g PRO; 4g Fiber

1   tablespoon extra virgin olive oil
1   cup chopped onion
2   garlic cloves, minced
2   cups *Basic Meat Sauce* (p 132)
1   25-ounce jar prepared pasta sauce
1   teaspoon Italian herb mix

In large skillet, heat olive oil over medium-high hea and sauté onion and garlic for 5 minutes. Add remaining ingredients and simmer uncovered for 20 minutes. Leftovers can be frozen for up to 3 months.

spaghetti with sauce

Serves 2
302 Calories per serving; 44g CHO; 6g FAT; 20g PRO; 9g Fiber

Heat 2 cups of *Sauce for Spaghetti or Lasagna* (p 133) or one 25-ounce jar purchased spaghetti sauce. Cook 3 ounces (about 1 cup uncooked) of whole grain pasta per manufacturer's directions and top with sauce. Sprinkle with 2 tablespoons grated Parmesan cheese (optional).

ENTRÉES

133

spaghetti squash spaghetti

Serves 2
318 Calories per serving; 39g CHO; 13g FAT; 16g PRO; 8g Fiber

1   tablespoon extra virgin olive oil
2   cups cooked spaghetti squash
1   cup sliced onions and mushrooms
1   garlic clove, minced
     sea salt and freshly-ground black pepper, to taste
2   cups *Sauce for Spaghetti or Lasagna* (p 133)
     Parmesan cheese (optional)

To cook the spaghetti squash, wash a whole squash and stab the thick skin of the squash several times so it can vent during cooking (otherwise, it could explode in the oven!). Place the whole squash on a cookie sheet in a 375° oven for 1 hour, turning every 15 minutes, until the skin is soft to the touch. Remove from the oven and let cool for 10-15 minutes. Slice squash open; scoop out and discard the seeds. With a fork, scrape the flesh, which will separate into strands. Measure the 2 cups for this recipe. (The remainder can be refrigerated for 2-3 days for another use.) Heat *Sauce for Spaghetti or Lasagna* in a saucepan. In a large skillet, heat olive oil over medium-high heat; sauté cooked spaghetti squash, onions, mushrooms and garlic for 5-7 minutes. Arrange vegetables on plates and top with sauce. Sprinkle with Parmesan, if desired.

zucchini "pasta"

Serves 2
296 Calories per serving; 35g CHO; 13g FAT; 17g PRO; 7g Fiber

1	tablespoon extra virgin olive oil
4	small zucchini
1	large onion, sliced
2	large garlic cloves, minced
	sea salt and freshly-ground black pepper, to taste
2	cups *Sauce for Spaghetti or Lasagna* (p 133
	grated Parmesan cheese (optional)

Slice unpeeled zucchini into ribbons lengthwise, using a vegetable peeler and turning the squash as you go. Stop slicing when you get to the center seed portion and discard remainder. (The seed portion gets very watery and mushy when sautéed.) Heat oil in a large skillet over medium-high heat; sauté onion, squash and garlic for 5 minutes until squash is soft and edges are clear. Add salt and pepper. Transfer mixture to individual serving plates and top with *Sauce for Spaghetti or Lasagna*. Sprinkle with Parmesan cheese, if desired.

ENTRÉES

135

zucchini "lasagna"

Serves 4
325 Calories per serving; 27g CHO; 13g FAT; 27g PRO; 6g Fiber

1	pound zucchini (about 3 medium)
½	teaspoon freshly-ground black pepper
1	tablespoon extra virgin olive oil, divided
2	medium onions, chopped
2	garlic cloves, minced
3	cups *Sauce for Spaghetti or Lasagna* (p 133)
1	cup low-fat cottage cheese or ricotta cheese
1	egg white (free-range), slightly beaten
2	tablespoons grated Parmesan cheese
1	cup (4 ounces) shredded part-skim mozzarella cheese

Preheat oven to 450 °, with rack at the bottom. Coat a large cookie sheet with extra virgin olive oil. To make zucchini "noodles," wash zucchini and cut ends off; cut lengthwise into ½-inch thick slices. Arrange zucchini slices on cookie sheet; sprinkle with pepper and ½ tablespoon olive oil. Roast for 10 minutes. Turn slices over and roast for an additional 5 minutes or until tender and nicely browned. Remove pan from oven and set aside. Reduce oven temperature to 350°.

Sauce: In a large skillet, heat ½ tablespoon olive oil over medium-high heat; sauté onion and garlic. Add *Sauce for Spaghetti or Lasagna.* Simmer uncovered a few minutes to thicken. Remove from heat and set aside. **Filling:** In a medium bowl, combine cottage cheese and egg white; stir to mix. Set aside.

To assemble lasagna, brush a 9x13-inch glass baking dish with oil. Add a thin layer of sauce just to cover the bottom. Layer half of the zucchini slices, sprinkle with 1 tablespoon Parmesan. Add half of remaining sauce and spread on all of the cottage cheese filling. Arrange remaining zucchini slices on top of filling. Cover with remaining 1 tablespoon Parmesan and remaining sauce. Bake uncovered for 20 minutes. Sprinkle mozzarella cheese over the top and bake for an additional 10 minutes or until the edges are bubbly and the cheese is melted and just starting to brown. Remove the dish from the oven and let it rest for 15 minutes before serving. Cut into squares and lift out with a spatula.

traditional lasagna

Set oven temperature to 350°. Follow the recipe for *Zucchini "Lasagna,"* using
6 whole grain lasagna noodles (cooked according to package directions) in place of
the zucchini "noodles."

spanish rice

6 cups
1 cup = 250 Calories; 37g CHO; 7g FAT; 11g PRO; 6g Fiber

2 tablespoons extra virgin olive oil
1 cup uncooked brown rice
½ green pepper, chopped
1 cup chopped onion
1 cup chopped mushrooms
2 cups **Basic Meat Sauce** (p 132)
1 14.5-ounce can Italian stewed tomatoes
1 cup tomato juice
1½ cups water
2 garlic cloves, minced
1½ teaspoons chili powder
1½ teaspoons mustard
½ teaspoon cumin
sea salt and freshly-ground black pepper, to taste

Heat olive oil over medium-high heat in a large skillet; sauté rice, green pepper,
onion, and mushrooms for 5 minutes. Add remaining ingredients and bring to a
boil. Cover (do not peek, or the rice could get gummy), reduce heat to very low and
simmer for 45-50 minutes.

ENTRÉES

137

goulash

Serves 3
330 Calories per serving; 42g CHO; 8g FAT; 26g PRO; 5g Fiber

1	tablespoon extra virgin olive oil
1	cup onion, chopped
¼	cup chopped green/red pepper
½	cup chopped mushrooms
1	garlic clove, minced
2	cups *Basic Meat Sauce* (p 132)
1	14.5-ounce can tomato juice
2	cups chicken broth
¾	cup uncooked whole grain macaroni
½	teaspoon chili powder

In large skillet, heat olive oil over medium-high heat; sauté onion, pepper, mushrooms, and garlic for 5 minutes. Add remaining ingredients. Simmer uncovered for 15-20 minutes.

barbecued pork or beef tenderloin

Serves 4
338 Calories per serving; 34g CHO; 6g FAT; 37g PRO; 3g Fiber

1½	pounds pork or beef tenderloin
	Barbecue sauce
4	tablespoons unsweetened natural applesauce
	dash of cinnamon
2-3	cups *Steamed Brown Rice* (p 175)

Grill tenderloin until meat is no longer pink (approximately 5 minutes on each of four sides). Brush tenderloin with barbecue sauce after the third turn. Remove from the grill; make an aluminum foil tent over it and let rest for 5 minutes before carving, to set the juices. Slice the meat thinly. Divide into 4 portions, top each with applesauce and sprinkle with cinnamon. Serve over ½-⅔ cup *Steamed Brown Rice.*

pork loin chops and peppers

Serves 6
312 Calories per serving; 13g CHO 16g FAT; 29g PRO; 2g Fiber

2   tablespoons extra virgin olive oil, divided
6   pork loin chops
    sea salt and freshly-ground black pepper to taste
¼   teaspoon dried rosemary, crushed
1   onion, sliced
¼   cup water
¼   cup whole wheat flour
2   cups soy milk
8   ounces mushrooms, sliced
1   green bell pepper, sliced into long thin strips
1   red bell pepper, sliced into long thin strips

Season chops with salt, pepper and rosemary. Heat 1 tablespoon oil in large skillet over medium-high heat; add chops and brown on both sides. Reduce temperature to simmer; add onion and water. Cover and cook slowly for 15 minutes. Remove chops and onion from skillet and set aside. Drain any liquid remaining in the skillet into a measuring cup and set aside. To prepare cream sauce, heat 1 tablespoon oil in skillet over medium heat, add mushrooms and peppers and sauté for 5 minutes. Add flour and stir. Add milk to liquid in measuring cup to equal 2 cups. Add to liquids to skillet and stir until thickened. Return chops to skillet and spoon sauce and vegetables over them. Cover and simmer 5 more minutes.

ENTRÉES

139

🌹 pan-seared chicken

Serves 2
190 Calories per serving; 0g CHO; 12 g FAT; 26g PRO; 0 Fiber

8   ounces boneless, skinless chicken breast
½   teaspoon lemon pepper
1   tablespoon extra virgin olive oil

Sprinkle chicken with seasonings and place between 2 layers of plastic wrap or waxed paper. With the flat side of a meat tenderizer, gently pound the thickest part of the breast so the overall thickness is uniform. In a large skillet, heat olive oil on medium. Add chicken pieces in a single layer and cook without moving them—2 minutes if tenders, 3 minutes if larger pieces. Turn the chicken with a metal spatula and cook 2-4 minutes more, depending on the size of the pieces. Remove to serving plates.

Variations: Replace lemon-pepper with one of these seasoning mixtures.

- *Taco Seasoning* (p 79)
- *Herbes de Provence* (p 79), sea salt, freshly-ground black pepper
- Italian herbs, sea salt, freshly-ground black pepper

chicken with snow peas

Serves 2-3
303 Calories per serving; 19g CHO; 14g FAT; 29g PRO; 6g Fiber

8   ounces boneless, skinless chicken breast
2   carrots, thinly sliced
¼   pound snow pea pods
1   tablespoon extra virgin olive oil, divided
6   slices gingerroot
1   can water chestnuts, drained
3   tablespoons chicken broth
1   teaspoon arrowroot

Marinade

1   teaspoon rice wine
½   teaspoon sea salt
½   teaspoon arrowroot

Seasoning Sauce

1   tablespoon rice wine
½   teaspoon sea salt
¼   teaspoon freshly-ground black pepper
1   teaspoon rice vinegar
1   teaspoon sesame oil

Cut chicken into thin slices (this is easier if chicken is still partially frozen), then into bite-size pieces. Mix marinade ingredients in a medium bowl; add chicken pieces, mix well. Let stand 20 minutes. Meanwhile, mix ingredients for seasoning sauce in small bowl and set aside. Heat half of the olive oil in large skillet or wok over medium heat. Stir-fry gingerroot for about 30 seconds; remove and discard. Add carrots and snow pea pods to oil and stir-fry for 2 minutes. Add water chestnuts and heat through. Remove vegetables from skillet and set aside. Heat remaining oil in same skillet over medium heat. Add chicken and stir-fry about 2 minutes. Add cooked vegetables; stir in seasoning sauce. Stir until sauce thickens slightly.

chicken stir-fry

Serves 4
236 Calories per serving; 10g CHO; 8g FAT; 31g PRO; 3g Fiber

- 1   pound boneless, skinless chicken breast
- 1   tablespoon extra virgin olive oil, divided
- 1   cup sliced carrots
- 1   cup sliced mushrooms
- 2   cups shredded cabbage
- 1   cup fresh bean sprouts
- 1   tablespoon reduced-sodium soy sauce
- 3   tablespoons natural peanut butter

Steam or sauté chicken in large skillet using half of the olive oil. Cut chicken into bite-size pieces and set aside. Stir-fry vegetables in remaining oil to desired tenderness. Add cooked chicken pieces to vegetables. Stir in peanut butter and soy sauce and heat through.

MJ's chicken stir-fry

4 servings
385 Calories per serving; 45g CHO; 8g FAT; 35g PRO; 7g Fiber

1   tablespoon extra virgin olive oil
1   pound boneless, skinless chicken breast, cut into 1-inch pieces
1   red, green or yellow pepper, sliced
1   pound fresh asparagus or broccoli, cut into 1-inch pieces
1   onion, sliced
3   tablespoons of your favorite stir-fry sauce (no hydrogenated fats or high fructose corn syrup)
1   tablespoon sesame teriyaki sauce (optional)
1   cup mixed wild rice

Cook rice according to package instructions. Heat olive oil in stir-fry pan; brown chicken (about 3 minutes). Add peppers, asparagus or broccoli and onion. Stir-fry until vegetables are tender (2-3 minutes). Stir in sauces and let cook for 5 more minutes. Serve over rice.

ENTRÉES

143

chicken fried rice

3 servings
366 Calories per serving; 31g CHO; 15g FAT; 28g PRO; 4g Fiber

2 tablespoons extra virgin coconut oil
1 cup chopped onion
1 cup chopped fresh mushrooms (button, shiitake, and/or Portobello)
½ cup snow pea pods, sliced diagonally
½ cup carrot, julienned
1 cup brown rice, cooked, cold
8 ounces cooked chicken, shredded
1 can water chestnuts, drained and chopped
½ teaspoon unrefined toasted sesame oil
2 tablespoons reduced-sodium soy sauce

In large skillet, heat oil over medium-high heat; sauté onions and mushrooms for 5 minutes. Add snow peas and carrots and sauté another 3-5 minutes. Add rice and sauté another 5 minutes. Add chicken and water chestnuts and heat through. Add sesame oil and soy sauce and stir.

orange chicken and rice

Serves 4
362 Calories per serving; 42g CHO; 9g FAT; 31g PRO; 3g Fiber

1   pound boneless, skinless chicken breast, cut into 2-inch pieces
1-2 tablespoons extra virgin olive oil
1   medium onion, coarsely chopped
1½ cups orange juice
1   14-ounce can chicken broth
1   cup whole grain rice, uncooked
2   garlic cloves, minced
⅓   teaspoon curry powder
     dash of cinnamon
3   tablespoons raisins (optional)
     sea salt and freshly-ground black pepper, to taste

In a large skillet, heat oil over medium-high heat; sauté chicken and onion until browned. Add orange juice, broth, rice, garlic and seasonings. Reduce heat, cover and simmer for 25 minutes. Add raisins (optional) to skillet and simmer 25 minutes or until rice is done (check the package for cooking time). Add more water or broth if the sauce gets too thick. Add salt and pepper to taste.

ENTRÉES   145

Carol's pineapple chicken

Serves 2
329 Calories per serving; 26g CHO; 14g FAT; 31g PRO; 5g Fiber

8   ounces boneless, skinless chicken breast, cut in 1-inch strips
    sea salt and freshly-ground black pepper, to taste
½   fresh pineapple (about 1½ cups), cut into chunks and gently pressed
    to extract about ¼ cup juice (set aside)
1   tablespoon extra virgin coconut oil
1   cup sliced onions
½   cup green pepper chunks
1   cup snow pea pods
2   cups sliced fresh button, shiitake or Portobello mushrooms
¼   cup julienned carrots
2   tablespoons lower-sodium soy sauce
1   teaspoon rice vinegar
1   teaspoon toasted sesame oil

Heat coconut oil in large skillet over medium heat. Add chicken strips and sauté for 5 minutes. Add onions, pepper, pea pods, mushrooms, carrots, and pineapple chunks and sauté an additional 2-3 minutes. In a small bowl, mix together the extracted pineapple juice, soy sauce, rice vinegar and sesame oil; add to the skillet and heat through. Serve with *Steamed Brown Rice* (p 175), one of the *Fried Rice* variations (p 175, 176), or *Mushroom Pilaf* (p 176).

poached chicken

Serves 4
155 Calories per serving; 5g CHO; 4g FAT; 27g PRO; 2g Fiber

2 cups chicken broth
2 stalks celery, chopped
2 carrots, chopped
1 medium onion, chopped
2 teaspoons dried tarragon
½ teaspoon sea salt
⅛ teaspoon freshly-ground black pepper
1 pound boneless, skinless chicken breast

In large saucepan, combine chicken broth, vegetables, tarragon, salt and pepper. Bring to a boil, add chicken, cover and simmer 10-15 minutes until chicken juices run clear. Remove the chicken with a slotted spoon. Thicken the sauce with 1 tablespoon arrowroot and serve over the chicken, or cool the chicken for use in soup, salad or sandwich recipes which call for cooked chicken (*Taco Salad, Chicken Salad, Cherry Chicken Salad, Chicken Waldorf Salad, Chicken Caesar Salad, White Chicken Chili, Quick Chicken Chili,* and *Chicken Salad Sandwich Filling* (see Index for page numbers).

ENTRÉES

147

chicken parmesan

Serves 4
478 Calories per serving; 52g CHO; 15g FAT; 36g PRO; 9g Fiber

A great company dish!

Tomato Sauce (or use 1 25-ounce jar of prepared spaghetti sauce)

1   tablespoon extra virgin olive oil
4   medium cloves garlic, minced
1   cup chopped onion
2   14.5-ounce cans crushed tomatoes
1   tablespoon balsamic vinegar
    sea salt and freshly-ground black pepper, to taste
2   tablespoons chopped fresh basil (1 teaspoon dried)
¼   cup chopped fresh Italian flat leaf parsley

12 ounces boneless, skinless chicken breast
1   egg (free-range), slightly beaten
    sea salt and freshly-ground black pepper, to taste
½   cup **Whole Grain Bread Crumbs** (p 51) mixed with 1 teaspoon Italian seasoning
1   tablespoon extra virgin olive oil
6   ounces whole wheat capellini or spaghetti
2   ounces (½ cup) grated Parmesan cheese

To prepare sauce, sauté garlic and onions in oil for 5 minutes over medium heat. Add tomatoes, vinegar, salt and pepper; simmer for 10-15 minutes, adding basil and parsley for last 3-5 minutes. (If using prepared spaghetti sauce, pour entire jar into skillet and heat through.) Meanwhile, flatten chicken breasts to ¼ inch. Dip each flattened chicken fillet into beaten egg, then into the bread crumbs. Heat olive oil in large skillet and add fillets in a single layer. Cook 2-3 minutes on each side or until golden brown. Preheat oven to 350°. Brush a 9x13-inch pan with olive oil. Spread a thin coat of tomato sauce in the bottom of the pan; arrange chicken on top. Put a small amount of tomato sauce on each fillet, reserving the remaining sauce. Sprinkle with grated Parmesan. Bake for 10-15 minutes. In a large saucepan, bring 5 quarts of water to a boil; add salt. Add pasta and cook according to package; drain and place in a serving bowl. Pour the remaining sauce over the pasta. Arrange the oven-cooked chicken on top of the pasta; serve.

nachos

Serves 4
¼ = 352 Calories; 48g CHO; 14g FAT; 17g PRO; 8g Fiber

4 ounces ground turkey, venison or buffalo
1 teaspoon extra virgin olive oil
2 tablespoons *Taco Seasoning* (p 79) mixed with ½ cup water
2 cups *Bean Dip* (p 77) or *Refried Beans* (p 179)
    or 1 15-ounce can fat-free refried beans
4 ounces blue corn chips made with expeller pressed canola oil or high oleic
    safflower oil
2 ounces (½ cup) shredded low-fat cheese
    tomato, onion, and avocado, all chopped
    salsa

In a large skillet, heat olive oil over medium-high heat and brown meat. Add seasoning and beans and warm through. Place chips on a cookie sheet. Top with the meat/bean mixture and sprinkle with cheese. Place the cookie sheet about 5 inches from the broiler and broil until the cheese melts. (Watch carefully, so it doesn't burn.) Sprinkle with the fresh vegetables; divide into portions; dip in salsa. YUM!

ENTRÉES

149

chicken fajitas

Serves 2
338 Calories per serving; 40g CHO; 15g FAT; 34g PRO; 9g Fiber (not including marinade)

2   tablespoons Italian dressing (made with extra virgin olive oil)
6   ounces boneless, skinless chicken breast
1   tablespoon extra virgin olive oil
1   tablespoon *Taco Seasoning* (p 79)
     dash of hot pepper sauce
1   small green bell pepper, cut in strips
1   small red bell pepper, cut in strips
1   medium onion, sliced
     freshly-ground black pepper
1   teaspoon paprika
2   tablespoons lime juice
1   tomato, diced
1   cup lshredded ettuce
1   avocado, sliced or chopped
4   6-inch whole wheat flour tortillas
½   cup salsa

ENTRÉES

Put dressing in a small zip top bag. Cut the chicken into ½-inch thick strips (this is easiest to do if the chicken is still partially-frozen) and add to the bag of dressing. Gently shake bag to make sure dressing coats all chicken pieces. Marinate 2 to 24 hours. Drain the chicken and discard the marinade. In a large skillet, heat olive oil over medium-high heat; add the drained chicken strips, **Taco Seasoning** and hot pepper sauce; sauté for 2 minutes. Add green and red pepper, onion, black pepper and paprika; sauté an additional 3-5 minutes until vegetables are tender. Remove skillet from heat. Sprinkle the meat mixture with the lime juice. Divide the meat mixture among the 4 tortillas. Top with the fresh vegetables and salsa.

🌹 easy cookie sheet dinner

Serves 2
370 Calories per serving; 41g CHO; 12g FAT; 33g PRO; 7g Fiber

1 large sweet potato, peeled and cut into ½-inch slices
1 tablespoon extra virgin olive oil, divided
8 ounces boneless, skinless chicken breast
½ teaspoon lemon pepper
8 ounces (combined) cleaned asparagus, green beans, onions, mushrooms and/or other preferred vegetables

Preheat oven to 425°. Lightly coat cookie sheet with some olive oil. Place sweet potato slices on cookie sheet in a single layer; sprinkle with 1 teaspoon of olive oil. Place cookie sheet on bottom rack in oven and roast for 10 minutes. Turn the potato slices over. Sprinkle chicken breast with lemon pepper. Place on the cookie sheet with the potato slices and drizzle with 1 teaspoon of olive oil; roast for an additional 10 minutes. Turn chicken pieces over and check potato slices for browning. Place vegetables on the cookie sheet with potato slices and chicken. Drizzle with 1 teaspoon of olive oil; roast for an additional 10 minutes. Shake the cookie sheet periodically after adding the vegetables to insure that they don't get overly browned on one side.

ENTRÉES 151

chicken tenders

Serves 4
255 Calories per serving; 17g CHO; 9g FAT; 31g PRO; 3g Fiber

| 1 | pound boneless, skinless chicken breast, cut in thirds
| | sea salt and freshly-ground black pepper, to taste
| 1 | cup *Whole Grain Bread Crumbs* (p 51)
| ½ | teaspoon dried thyme or poultry seasoning
| ½ | teaspoon garlic powder
| 6 | ounces low-fat plain or lemon yogurt
| 1 | tablespoon extra virgin olive oil

Place chicken pieces between 2 pieces of plastic wrap and pound the thickest part of the chicken breast with the flat side of a meat tenderizer to flatten. Season chicken with salt and pepper. Combine bread crumbs and seasonings on a plate; put yogurt on another plate. Dredge chicken through yogurt, shake off excess, dredge in crumbs, and shake off excess. Heat olive oil in a large skillet over medium-high heat; brown dredged chicken pieces for 4-5 minutes on each side, turning once with a metal spatula.

no-fry chicken

Serves 4
270 Calories per serving; 21g CHO; 8g FAT; 30g PRO; 2g Fiber

  4   boneless, skinless chicken breast halves
  ¾   cup plain non-fat yogurt
  1   tablespoon spicy mustard
  ½   cup *Whole Grain Bread Crumbs* (p 51)
  ½   cup whole grain flour (unbleached, unbromated)
  1   tablespoon extra virgin olive oil

Preheat oven to 400°. Lightly coat a cookie sheet with extra virgin olive oil. Cool chicken in ice water; remove and pat dry with paper towel. Combine yogurt and mustard in a small bowl. Combine bread crumbs and flour in another small bowl. Dip chicken in yogurt mixture then roll in bread crumb mixture. Place on oiled cookie sheet. Bake 30-40 minutes or until cooked through, turning after 15 minutes to brown bottom.

ENTRÉES

153

oven-fried chicken

Serves 4
199 Calories per serving; 17g CHO; 9g FAT; 31g PRO; 3g Fiber

1	pound boneless, skinless chicken breast
¾	cup skim milk
⅓	cup *Whole Grain Bread Crumbs* (p 51)
½	teaspoon dried thyme, sage, and/or poultry seasoning
½	teaspoon garlic powder
½	teaspoon paprika
⅛	teaspoon ground black pepper
1	tablespoon extra virgin olive oil

Preheat oven to 450°. Rinse and pat chicken dry. Soak chicken in skim milk in refrigerator for 30 minutes. In small bowl, mix bread crumbs, herbs, and pepper. Drain chicken. Dip in bread crumbs. Place on a wire cooling rack over a cookie sheet and refrigerate for 30 minutes. (This helps the chicken become crispy all around.) Sprinkle chicken lightly with olive oil. Bake on the wire cooling rack over the cookie sheet for 20 minutes.

yogurt chicken

Serves 7
226 Calories per serving; 5g CHO; 10g FAT; 29g PRO; < 1g Fiber

2   pounds skinless chicken thighs (bone-in)
2   tablespoons lemon or lime juice
1   tablespoon extra virgin olive oil
1   cup plain low-fat yogurt
3   tablespoons canola mayonnaise
1   tablespoon Dijon mustard
1   tablespoon Worcestershire sauce
½   teaspoon dried thyme
¼   cup sliced green onion (including green tops)
¼   teaspoon cayenne pepper or to taste
¼   cup Parmesan cheese, grated

Preheat oven to 350°. Arrange chicken pieces in a shallow baking dish. In a small bowl, blend juice and oil together; pour over chicken. Bake uncovered for approximately 50 minutes. Remove from oven and drain off all accumulated juices. In a small bowl, blend together yogurt, mayonnaise, mustard, Worcestershire sauce, thyme, onion and pepper; spread over chicken. Sprinkle with Parmesan cheese. Return pan to oven and broil until cheese melts and begins to brown.

ENTRÉES

155

chicken cordon bleu

Serves 2
295 Calories per serving; 14g CHO; 10g FAT; 39g PRO; 2g Fiber

A great company dish!

2   4-ounce boneless, skinless chicken cutlets (or flattened chicken breast)
2   1-ounce slices turkey ham (non-cured, nitrate-free)
2   slices low-fat swiss cheese
1½ tablespoons Dijon mustard, divided
1   teaspoon honey
⅓   cup **Whole Grain Bread Crumbs** (p 51)
1   cup chicken broth
2   teaspoons whole wheat flour (unbleached, unbromated)
½   teaspoon dried French tarragon
1   tablespoon low-fat sour cream

Preheat the oven to 375°. Lay each cutlet flat on a plate. (If using chicken breast, place each breast between two sheets of plastic wrap and gently pound with the flat side of a meat tenderizer to flatten.) Top each cutlet with a slice of ham, then a slice of cheese. Roll up and secure with toothpick or metal skewer.
In a small bowl, combine honey and 1 tablespoon of mustard. Spread mixture over chicken rolls. Sprinkle bread crumbs on a plate; roll each chicken bundle in the crumbs. Place on a cookie sheet or small roasting pan that has been brushed with olive oil. Sprinkle olive oil on the chicken bundles and bake until chicken is cooked through, about 20-25 minutes. While the chicken is cooking, combine broth, tarragon and flour in small saucepan, stirring until the flour dissolves. Cook over medium heat, stirring often until sauce thickens, about 3-4 minutes. Reduce heat to low and stir in low-fat sour cream and remaining mustard. Cook an additional 3-4 minutes on low. **Do not boil.** Remove toothpicks. Pour sauce over chicken and serve.

chicken in a packet

Serves 4
242 Calories per serving; 15g CHO; 10g FAT; 30g PRO; 5g Fiber

1   pound boneless, skinless chicken breast
1   tablespoon extra virgin olive oil
1   teaspoon lemon pepper
2   teaspoons garlic and herb seasoning
4   cups sliced fresh mushrooms
2   onions, quartered
1   medium zucchini, cut into 1-inch chunks
4   medium carrots, cut into julienne strips

Preheat oven to 375°. Fold 4 pieces of heavy duty aluminum foil to make four 18x12-inch rectangles. Place 1 chicken breast on each piece of foil, tucking under thin tip of chicken. Fold up edges of foil slightly. In a small bowl, mix oil and seasonings. Drizzle over chicken. Top with vegetables, dividing them evenly among bundles. Fold foil around each chicken bundle securely. Place on a cookie sheet or shallow baking pan. Bake for 30-35 minutes. Open packets carefully to avoid steam burn.

ENTRÉES

157

Mary's chicken and rice casserole

Serves 2
393 Calories per serving; 42g CHO; 13g FAT; 30g PRO; 6g Fiber

4	teaspoons extra virgin coconut oil, divided
½	cup each chopped celery, onion, mushrooms
½	cup uncooked brown rice
¼	fresh pineapple chunks
½	teaspoon sea salt
	freshly-ground black pepper
¼	teaspoon poultry seasoning
1½	teaspoon lower-sodium soy sauce
1¾	cups chicken broth
8	ounces boneless, skinless chicken breast

Preheat oven to 350°. Heat 1 teaspoon coconut oil in a large skillet over medium heat. Sauté chopped vegetables for 5 minutes, remove from pan to a bowl and set aside. In same skillet, heat 1 teaspoon coconut oil; add rice, sauté for 2 minutes then add sautéed vegetables, pineapple, salt, pepper, poultry seasoning, soy sauce, and chicken broth. Heat to boiling, pour into oiled 1½-quart casserole and cover. Bake for 1 hour. Brown chicken in remaining 2 teaspoons coconut oil in fry pan and add to casserole. Push the chicken down into the rice, cover and bake for 15 more minutes, leaving uncovered so sauce can thicken.

baked chicken and vegetables

Serves 4
304 Calories per serving; 36g CHO; 4g FAT; 31g PRO; 6g Fiber

4	carrots, sliced thick
2	large redskin potatoes, sliced thick
2	medium sweet potatoes, sliced thick
4	boneless, skinless chicken breast halves
	sea salt and freshly-ground black pepper, to taste
	sprinkle of garlic powder
½	teaspoon dried thyme
2	yellow onions, sliced thin
1½	cups chicken broth
⅛	cup almonds, slivered

Preheat oven to 350°. Line bottom of a large casserole dish with carrots and potato slices. Place chicken breasts on top and sprinkle with seasonings. Cover with onion slices. Pour broth or water over ingredients. Cover and bake for 90 minutes until tender. Sprinkle almonds on top and serve.

oven roasted whole chicken

Serves 4
4 ounces chicken + ¼ of vegetables = 336 Calories; 23g CHO; 10g FAT; 38g PRO; 3g Fiber

1	4-pound broiler chicken
2	garlic cloves, minced
1	tablespoon extra virgin olive oil
½	teaspoon dried thyme
½	teaspoon dried rosemary
¼	teaspoon sea salt
	freshly-ground black pepper
1	stalk celery, cut in chunks
2	medium onions, quartered
1	lemon, quartered
	sprig of fresh rosemary, if available
2	medium unpeeled, redskin potatoes, halved lengthwise
4	medium carrots, peeled and quartered
½	cup water

Preheat oven to 400°. Rinse chicken and pat dry with paper towel; place in a clay baker, breast side up. In a small bowl, combine garlic, oil, thyme, rosemary, salt and pepper and rub under breast skin and over chicken. Stuff cavity with celery, onion, lemon and fresh rosemary. Tuck potato and carrots around chicken. Pour water around chicken. Cover and bake 90 minutes or until thermometer inserted in breast meat reads 170°. Remove lid during last 20 minutes of baking to allow chicken to brown. Remove chicken from oven and cover with tented aluminum foil. Let chicken rest 10 minutes before carving so juices will set.

chicken and vegetable kebabs

Serves 6
183 Calories per serving; 2g CHO; 9g FAT; 27g PRO; 1g Fiber (not including marinade)

¼   cup fresh lemon juice
2   tablespoons chopped fresh oregano
2   tablespoons extra virgin olive oil
1½ pounds boneless, skinless chicken breast, cut into 24 strips
18   slices zucchini, sliced ½-inch thick
12   large garlic cloves
½   teaspoon sea salt
¼   teaspoon freshly-ground black pepper

Combine lemon juice, oregano, olive oil, chicken, and zucchini in zip-top plastic bag; seal and shake well. Set bag in refrigerator to marinate for at least 20 minutes. Cook garlic cloves in boiling water for 3 minutes; drain and cool. Remove chicken mixture from bag and discard marinade. Thread 4 chicken strips, 3 zucchini slices and 2 garlic cloves alternately onto each of 6 skewers. (If using bamboo skewers, be sure to soak them in water for 20 minutes before making the kebabs to prevent burning.) Sprinkle with salt and pepper. Brush grill with olive oil to prevent sticking. Grill kebabs for 8 minutes, turning once, or until chicken is done.

Variation: Brush kebabs with salsa after first turn.

ENTRÉES

161

baked eggplant

Serves 6
210 Calories per serving; 27g CHO; 2g FAT; 21g PRO; 6g Fiber (not including rice)

1	tablespoon extra virgin olive oil
1	pound lean ground turkey
2	medium onions, chopped
½	teaspoon sea salt
½	teaspoon freshly-ground black pepper
½	teaspoon ground allspice
½	teaspoon cinnamon
3	large eggplants, peeled and cut into 1/2-inch slices
1	15-ounce can tomato puree
3	cups *Steamed Brown Rice* (p 175)

In large skillet, heat olive oil over medium heat and brown turkey, stirring to separate meat particles. A onion and seasonings, sauté an additional 5 minutes and set aside. Broil or sauté eggplant in large skillet until tender. Preheat oven to 375°. In a 9x13-inch pan, layer eggplant then turkey mixture. Pour tomato puree over all. Bake for 20-25 minutes or until bubbly. Serve over ½ cup *Steamed Brown Rice*.

pan-seared fish

Serves 2
214 Calories per serving; 1g CHO; 12g FAT; 26g PRO; 0g Fiber

10 ounces cod fillets, thawed
 2 tablespoons lemon juice
1½ tablespoons extra virgin olive oil
     lemon pepper

Rinse fish well in cold water and pat dry with paper towels. Sprinkle with lemon juice, then lemon pepper. Over medium heat, heat the olive oil in a large skillet. Add fish in a single layer and cook without moving for 4 minutes. Turn fish over with a metal spatula and cook for 2-4 minutes more, depending on the thickness of the fish, until the fish flakes easily with a fork. Serve with *Tartar Sauce* (p 78).

fish fingers

4 servings
141 Calories per serving; 17g CHO; 1g FAT; 23g PRO; 1g Fiber

1	pound frozen cod, partially thawed, cut in 1-inch strips
½	low-fat plain or lemon yogurt
½	cup **Whole Grain Bread Crumbs** (p 51)
1	tablespoon grated lemon peel
¼	teaspoon lemon pepper
½	teaspoon paprika
½	teaspoon dried thyme
¼	teaspoon garlic powder

Preheat oven to 425°. Put yogurt on a plate. Combine bread crumbs and seasonings on another plate. Dip fish into yogurt then bread crumb mixture, shaking off excess. Place on a wire cooling rack over a cookie sheet and refrigerate for 20 minutes. (This helps the fish become crispy all around.) Bake for 15 minutes. Let stand for 2 minutes. Serve with *Tartar Sauce* (p 78). For a complete meal, start by adding *Roasted Sweet Potato Wedges* (p 189) to the cookie sheet for the first 15 minutes; then add the fish for 5 more minutes; then add your choice of vegetables for the last 10 minutes.

crispy cod

Serves 2
256 Calories per serving; 14g CHO; 9g FAT; 30g PRO; 1g Fiber

10	ounces cod fillet, thawed
1	egg white (free-range)
1	tablespoon water
½	cup **Whole Grain Bread Crumbs** (p 51)
2	tablespoons chopped Italian flat leaf parsley
½	teaspoon sea salt
¼	teaspoon lemon pepper
1	tablespoon extra virgin olive oil

Preheat oven to 400°. Brush an 8x8-inch pan with olive oil. In a small bowl, beat egg white and water. Dip fillets in egg white then roll in bread crumbs. Arrange fish in baking pan. Sprinkle with parsley, salt and lemon pepper and drizzle with olive oil. Bake uncovered 20 minutes or until fish flakes easily with a fork.

parmesan cod

Serves 2
220 Calories per serving; 0g CHO; 10g FAT; 28g PRO; 0g Fiber

10	ounces cod fillets, thawed
1	tablespoon lemon juice
	sea salt and freshly-ground black pepper, to taste
¼	cup canola mayonnaise
3	tablespoons Parmesan cheese
1	tablespoon thinly-sliced onion
⅛	teaspoon hot sauce

Preheat oven broiler. Brush broiler rack with olive oil and place cod on broiler rack. Sprinkle with lemon juice, salt and pepper. Mix remaining ingredients and spread on each fillet. Broil 5½ inches from the broiler until top is lightly browned and fish is flaky. Do not turn over.

salmon or tuna patties

Serves 4 or 5
274 Calories per serving; 16g CHO; 12g FAT; 26g PRO; 2g Fiber

1   16-ounce can salmon or tuna
1   teaspoon lemon juice
½   cup chopped onion
½   cup chopped celery
4   egg whites (free-range)
⅔   cup **Whole Grain Bread Crumbs** (p 51)
2   tablespoons soy milk
2   tablespoons extra virgin olive oil

Drain salmon or tuna. Discard bones and skin and flake meat. Combine fish
with lemon juice, onion, celery, egg whites, ⅓ cup bread crumbs and milk; mix
well. Shape into 4 or 5 patties and coat with remaining bread crumbs. In large
skillet, heat oil over medium heat. Cook patties about 3 minutes or until browned.
Carefully turn with metal spatula and brown other side about 3 minutes more.

grilled salmon and vegetables

Serves 4
292 Calories per serving; 10g CHO; 10g FAT; 37g PRO; 3g Fiber (excluding the marinade)

1½ pounds wild-caught salmon fillets
 1   eggplant, sliced ½-inch thick
4-5 large Portobello mushrooms, sliced
 1   red bell pepper, sliced

Marinade

⅓ cup expeller pressed canola oil
¼ cup lemon or lime juice
1-3 garlic cloves, minced
½ teaspoon paprika
½ teaspoon ground cumin

Mix marinade ingredients in large bowl or zip top bag. Add fish and vegetables, gently shake bag to coat all surfaces, and marinate for about 1 hour in the refrigerator. Remove fish and vegetables from marinade; discard marinade. Grill or broil salmon and vegetables until salmon flakes easily with a fork and vegetables are tender.

salmon teriyaki

Serves 6
216 Calories per serving; 6g CHO; 10g FAT; 27g PRO; 2g Fiber (excluding rice or potatoes)

2 pounds wild-caught salmon fillets
8 fresh green onions (including green tops), chopped
12 slices fresh gingerroot
½ cup light teriyaki sauce or Bragg's Liquid Aminos™
2 cups *Steamed Brown Rice* (p 175)

Preheat oven to 425°. Place salmon in shallow baking dish, skin side down. Sprinkle with onions, scatter gingerroot slices and pour teriyaki or Bragg's over the salmon. Cover tightly with aluminum foil. Bake 20 minutes or until fish flakes easily with a fork. Serve with ½ cup *Steamed Brown Rice* or 2 small redskin potatoes.

paprika-cumin salmon fillets

Serves 6
196 Calories per serving; 1g CHO; 9g FAT; 27g PRO; 0g Fiber

2 pounds skinned wild-caught salmon fillets, cut into 4 pieces
1 teaspoon extra virgin olive oil
1 teaspoon ground cumin
½ teaspoon sea salt
1 teaspoon paprika
½ teaspoon freshly-ground black pepper

In a large skillet, heat oil over medium heat. Combine spices and sprinkle on both sides of fish. Cook fish in a single layer for 4-5 minutes on each side, depending on the thickness of the fillets, or until the fish flakes easily with a fork.

salmon fillets in garlic

Serves 2
280 Calories per serving; 0g CHO; 17g FAT; 24g PRO; 0g Fiber

8   ounces wild-caught salmon fillet, skin on
      sea salt and freshly-ground black pepper, to taste
2   tablespoons Italian flat leaf parsley, snipped
2   tablespoons chicken broth
2   tablespoons dry white wine (or more chicken broth)
2   teaspoons extra virgin olive oil
2   large garlic cloves, minced
¼   teaspoon crushed red pepper

Preheat oven to 425°. Rinse salmon and pat dry with a paper towel. Sprinkle with salt and pepper. Place skin side down in 1½-quart casserole. Mix remaining ingredients in a bowl and pour evenly over salmon. Bake uncovered for 8-12 minutes until fish flakes easily.

ENTRÉES   169

baked salmon with mustard

Serves 2
308 Calories per serving; 7g CHO; 17g FAT; 26g PRO; 1g Fiber

8   ounces wild-caught salmon fillet, skin on
1   tablespoon balsamic vinegar
¾   teaspoon dry mustard
1   tablespoon Dijon mustard
2   teaspoons extra virgin olive oil
¼   cup *Whole Grain Bread Crumbs* (p 51)
½   teaspoon dried thyme
¼   teaspoon garlic powder
    sea salt

Preheat oven to 375°. Rinse and pat dry salmon. Sprinkle with salt and place skin side down in 1½ quart baking dish. Mix vinegar, mustards and olive oil until well blended. Spoon over each fillet, covering completely. Combine breadcrumbs with dried thyme and garlic powder. Press breadcrumbs onto fish. Bake until flaky, about 18 minutes.

🌹 pan-seared salmon

Serves 4
200 Calories per serving; 0g CHO; 11g FAT; 24g PRO; 0g Fiber

1 pound center-cut salmon fillet (skin on)
   sea salt and freshly-ground black pepper, to taste
2 teaspoons extra virgin olive oil

To insure even cooking, create pieces of salmon with equal thickness as follows: Lay the whole salmon fillet, skin side down, on a cutting board, with the length of the fillet going left to right. First cut the whole fillet into 3-inch wide pieces, cutting from the top to the bottom of fillet, through the skin. With each 3-inch piece, make a parallel cut down to, but not through, the skin. Insert a small metal skewer through the two halves to hold the pieces together during cooking.

Season fillets on both sides. Heat a large skillet over medium heat, add oil and fillets. Cook about 4½ minutes without moving the fillets. Turn the fillets and continue cooking another 3½ to 4 minutes. Remove the metal skewers, skin, bones and grayed flesh. Excellent in *Salmon Asparagus Chowder* (p 103) or in a *Taco Salad* (p 67).

ENTRÉES

171

shrimp with snow peas

Serves 4
240 Calories per serving; 13g CHO; 10g FAT; 26g PRO; 2g Fiber

1   pound raw, cleaned shrimp, shelled and deveined
2   tablespoons extra virgin olive oil, divided
3   cups snow peas, bok choy, and/or carrots
6-8 green onions, sliced
1   garlic clove, crushed

Marinade

1½ teaspoons rice wine (mirin)
½   teaspoon minced fresh gingerroot
1½ teaspoons arrowroot
1   teaspoon toasted sesame oil

Seasoning Sauce

1   tablespoon chicken broth
3   tablespoons water
1   teaspoon arrowroot
3   tablespoons oyster sauce

Combine marinade ingredients (rice wine, gingerroot, arrowroot, sesame oil) in medium bowl. Add shrimp and let stand 30 minutes. Drain marinade from shrimp, pat shrimp dry with a paper towel and set aside. Combine seasoning sauce ingredients (broth, water, arrowroot, oyster sauce) in small bowl; set aside. In large skillet or wok, heat 1 tablespoon olive oil over medium-high heat. Add snow peas, bok choy, carrots and green onions and stir-fry for 1-3 minutes. Remove to a bowl. Heat 1 tablespoon olive oil. Add garlic and shrimp and stir-fry for 1-2 minutes until shrimp are pink. Add seasoning sauce and stir until thickened. Add vegetables and stir to coat. Serve. Good with *Veggie Fried Rice* (p 176).

VEGETABLES AND SIDES

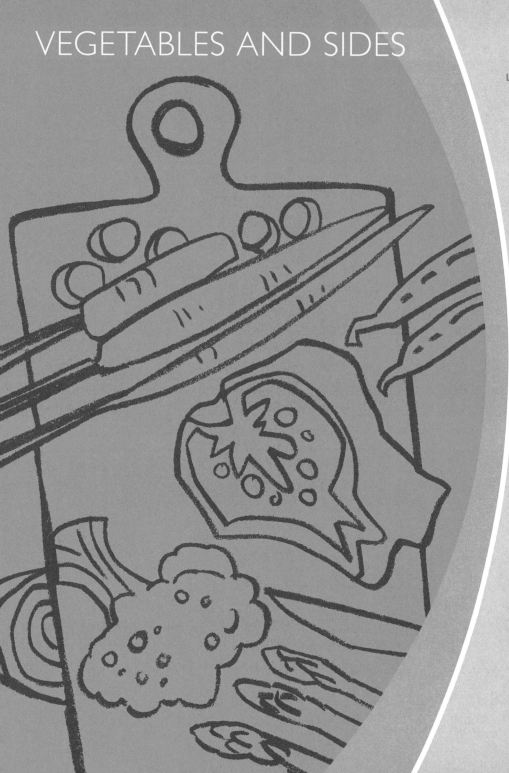

vegetables and sides

🌽 = Cook's Favorite

steamed brown rice

Makes 2½ cups
½ cup = 150 Calories; 32g CHO; 1g FAT; 3g PRO; 2g Fiber

Place 1 cup of long-grain brown rice in a medium saucepan. Add 2 cups of cold
water and a pinch of sea salt. Bring to a boil over high heat. Cover immediately
and turn to lowest heat setting; simmer for 50 minutes. Do not lift the cover
or the rice will become gummy. When the cooking time is up, uncover and fluff
rice with a fork. May be refrigerated for up to 3 days or frozen in a zip top bag for
up to 2 months.

basic fried rice

Serves 3
221 Calories per serving; 27g CHO; 12g FAT; 3g PRO; 3g Fiber

2   tablespoons extra virgin olive oil
1   cup chopped onion
1   cup chopped fresh mushrooms
1   cup long-grain brown rice, cooked, cold
1   teaspoon toasted sesame oil
1   tablespoon reduced-sodium soy sauce

In large skillet, heat olive oil over medium-high heat and sauté onions
and mushrooms for 5 minutes. Add cold rice and sauté another 5 minutes.
Add sesame oil and soy sauce and stir. Serve with *Grilled, Roasted, or
Stir-Fried Vegetables.*

VEGETABLES AND SIDES

175

veggie fried rice

3 servings
244 Calories per serving; 31g CHO; 13g FAT; 4g PRO; 7g Fiber

2	tablespoons extra virgin olive oil
1	garlic clove, minced
1	cup chopped onion
1	cup chopped fresh mushrooms
1½	cups broccoli slaw or chopped broccoli
½	cup chopped carrots
1	cup long-grain brown rice, cooked, cold
1	teaspoon toasted sesame oil
1	tablespoon reduced-sodium soy sauce

In large skillet, heat the olive oil over medium-high heat; sauté the garlic and onions for 5 minutes. Add the mushrooms, broccoli, and carrots and sauté another 5 minutes. Add the cold rice and sauté another 5 minutes. Add the sesame oil and soy sauce and stir. Serve.

mushroom pilaf

Serves 4
198 Calories per serving; 36g CHO; 6g FAT; 4g PRO; 3g Fiber

1	tablespoon extra virgin olive oil
½	large onion, chopped
1	cup mushrooms (button, shiitake, and/or Portobello), sliced
1	cup uncooked brown rice
2	cups chicken broth
½	teaspoon toasted sesame oil

In large skillet, heat olive oil and sauté onions and mushrooms for 5 minutes. Add rice and stir to coat grains with oil. Add chicken broth and sesame oil. Bring to a boil, cover, and reduce heat; simmer on very low heat for 50 minutes, or until all broth is absorbed. Do not lift cover until end of cooking time or the rice will become gummy.

asparagus and pasta stir-fry

Serves 4
209 Calories per serving; 33g CHO; 5g FAT; 9g PRO; 8g Fiber

6   ounces whole grain vermicelli, cooked and drained
½   teaspoon sea salt
2   teaspoons extra virgin olive oil
1   clove garlic, minced or pressed
1   teaspoon fresh minced gingerroot,
1   pound fresh asparagus, tough ends trimmed,
     cut diagonally into 1.5-inch pieces (about 3 cups)
1   cup diagonally-sliced green onions
2   tablespoons reduced-sodium soy sauce
1   teaspoon toasted sesame oil
⅛   teaspoon crushed red pepper flakes

In a large saucepan, bring 5 quarts of water to a boil; add salt and pasta
to cook while the remainder of the dish is prepared. In large skillet, heat
olive oil over medium heat; add garlic, gingerroot, asparagus and onions and
sauté for 3-5 minutes (depending on the size of the asparagus). Add soy sauce,
sesame oil and red pepper flakes and stir for 1 minute. Add the cooked pasta
and heat through.

Variation: Add 12 ounces of cooked shrimp or chicken to increase protein.

VEGETABLES AND SIDES

177

pasta with asparagus

Serves 4
340 Calories per serving; 50g CHO; 10g FAT; 15g PRO; 11g Fiber

8	ounces (about 2½ cups dry) whole grain penne or elbow macaroni
½	teaspoon sea salt
2	tablespoons extra virgin olive oil
5	garlic cloves, minced
1	onion, sliced
¼	teaspoon red pepper flakes
2-3	dashes hot pepper sauce
1	pound fresh asparagus, tough ends trimmed, cut into 1½-inch pieces (about 3 cups) sea salt and freshly-ground black pepper, to taste
1	14.5-ounce can Italian stewed tomatoes
¼	cup (1 ounce) shredded Parmesan cheese

In a large saucepan, bring 5 quarts of water to a boil; add salt and pasta to cook while the remainder of the dish is prepared. In a large skillet, heat olive oil over medium-high heat; add the garlic, onion, pepper flakes and hot pepper sauce and cook for 2-3 minutes. Add asparagus to the skillet, season with salt and pepper and sauté for 5-8 minutes. Add tomatoes and heat through. Drain the pasta and place it in a serving bowl. Pour the asparagus/tomato sauce over the pasta and sprinkle with Parmesan cheese.

refried beans

4 cups
½ cup = 165 Calories; 28g CHO; 5g FAT; 3g PRO; 7g Fiber

2   cups pinto beans, washed and picked over
4   cups water (for soaking)
5   cups water (for cooking)
2   tablespoons extra virgin olive oil
1   teaspoon crushed garlic
1   cup chopped onion
1-2   tablespoons *Taco Seasoning* (p 79)
⅛   teaspoon freshly-ground black pepper

Place beans and 4 cups of water in a large saucepan and let soak 6 hours or overnight. (Or, do a quick soak: boil the beans in 4 cups of water for 2 minutes; cover, let stand for 1 hour, and drain.) The next day (or right after completing the quick soak), return beans to the saucepan and add 5 cups of water. Bring to a boil, reduce heat and simmer until tender, 2-3 hours. Drain the beans, reserving some of the cooking liquid. In a large skillet, heat oil over medium-high heat and sauté garlic and onions for 5 minutes. Mash half of the beans and add to onion and garlic in the skillet. Continue to sauté for 10 minutes, stirring frequently. Allow some of the mashed beans to brown. Add *Taco Seasoning* and remaining beans and continue cooking until they are warmed through. Add water or the reserved cooking liquid as needed to keep the beans soft and creamy. Use in *Bean Dip* (p 77) and *Nachos* (p 149). Freezes well.

179

VEGETABLES AND SIDES

🌀 basic roasted vegetables

Nutritional values will vary depending on the selection and quantity of vegetables.

Preheat oven to 400° to 450°, depending on recipe. Use cookie sheet that has been coated liberally with extra virgin olive oil. Toss servings of a single vegetable or a combination of vegetables with additional extra virgin olive oil, sea salt, pepper, a handful of peeled, whole garlic cloves, and any other seasonings listed. Spread on cookie sheet in a single layer. Roast until tender and browned, **shaking pan at least once or turning vegetables during cooking to prevent burning.** Eat as is or season with sauce of choice. Leftovers are great on *Pita Pizza*, on salads or in *Stuffed Pita* (p 115).

VEGETABLE	PREP/MARINADE	TEMPERATURE/TIME
Asparagus	2 pounds asparagus, trimmed; I tablespoon extra virgin olive oil, sea salt, pepper. Proceed with general roasting directions.	425° 10-15 minutes
Beans, Green	I¼ pounds trimmed green beans, 2 tablespoons slivered almonds, I tablespoon lemon juice, 2 teaspoons extra virgin olive oil, ½ teaspoon sea salt, ¼ teaspoon garlic powder, ¼ teaspoon dried basil (I teaspoon fresh), freshly-ground black pepper. Proceed with general roasting directions.	450° 10 minutes
Broccoli or Cauliflower	I pound broccoli or cauliflower florets, 2 tablespoons extra virgin olive oil, 6-8 whole garlic cloves, sea salt, pepper in zip top bag; toss to coat. Spread I tablespoon olive oil on cookie sheet, add vegetable. Roast and then sprinkle with I tablespoon balsamic vinegar.	425° 20 minutes
Brussels Sprouts	I pound fresh Brussels sprouts (cut in half), 2 tablespoons extra virgin olive oil, sea salt in zip top bag; toss to coat. Spread I tablespoon olive oil on cookie sheet, add Brussels sprouts. Roast and then sprinkle with I tablespoon grated Parmesan cheese.	425° 15-20 minutes
Carrots, Parsnips and/or Rutabaga	Cut in uniform thick slices then prepare same as broccoli/cauliflower, omitting vinegar	425° 15 minutes
Mushrooms	Whole if small, sliced if portobellos. Proceed with general roasting directions.	425° 10-15 minutes
Onions	Cut in quarters or eighths, depending on size of onion. Proceed with general roasting directions.	425° 10-15 minutes
Potato (purple, redskin, sweet)	For *Roasted Redskin Potatoes* (p 190) or *Roasted Sweet Potato Wedges* (p 189)	
Squash (winter, butternut, acorn)	Cut squash lengthwise and scoop out the seeds. Then cut squash crosswise to make half-moons. Brush a cookie sheet with extra virgin olive oil. Lay squash on the cookie sheet. Brush with more olive oil; sprinkle with sea salt and pepper. Bake, turning once, until tender and golden.	400° 25-30 minutes
Squash (summer, zucchini)	Cut small to medium, unpeeled squash diagonally in ¼-inch slices. Proceed with general roasting directions.	425° 10-15 minutes
I pound assorted summer squash, I large bell pepper, 2 large onions	Cut squash into ½-inch slices, pepper into I-inch strips and onion in quarters. Put in zip top bag with marinade (I tablespoon balsamic or red wine vinegar, I tablespoon fresh basil, I tablespoon dried thyme, I teaspoon Dijon mustard, 2 tablespoons extra virgin olive oil) for I hour. Drain vegetables, discard marinade and proceed with general roasting directions.	425° 10-15 minutes
I bag frozen carrots/broccoli/cauliflower; I bunch asparagus;10 whole small cap mushrooms; 5 onions (quartered)	Drizzle with 3 tablespoons extra virgin olive oil, sea salt, pepper, garlic powder. Proceed with general roasting directions	400° 30 minutes

VEGETABLES AND SIDES

basic grilled vegetables

Nutritional values vary depending on the selection and quantity of vegetables.

General Directions: Blanch vegetables in boiling water, if indicated, and drain. Cut to recommended size. Brush vegetables with extra virgin olive oil, salt, pepper, herbs OR put vegetables in a zip top bag with one of the marinades listed on page 187 for 30 minutes to 24 hours, drain the vegetables and discard the marinade. Grill over moderately hot coals, and move to cooler part of the grill as necessary to finish. (It's helpful to use a holed vegetable grill on top of the grate to prevent the vegetables from slipping through.) Add one of the toppings listed on page 183, if desired.

VEGETABLES AND SIDES

VEGETABLE	PREP/MARINADE	BLANCH TIME	COOK TIME
Asparagus	whole spears		8-12 minutes
Carrots	2-inch chunks; halved lengthwise	3 minutes	10-15 minutes
Corn	remove silk; wet kernels or brush with extra virgin olive oil; grill in husk		15-20 minutes
Mushroom, Portobello Mushroom (canned) Mushrooms, small cap (button, crimini)	whole, slices, ¾-inch canned whole, fresh		12-20 minutes 10-12 minutes 5-6 minutes 6-10 minutes
Onions	sliced ¾-inch (horizontally), double skewer with toothpicks pre-soaked in water or metal skewers		10-15 minutes 10-15 minutes
Green Onion	whole		
Pepper, Green or Red	whole eighths		15-20 minutes 10-12 minutes
Potato, (purple, redskin)	2-3 inches in diameter, scrubbed, whole sliced ¾ inch thick	10 minutes 5 minutes	20-30 minutes 20-30 minutes
Sweet Potato			
Tomatoes	whole, 3-4 inches in diameter		15-18 minutes
Zucchini	⅜-inch lengthwise slices		8-12 minutes

marinades and toppings for basic grilled vegetables or basic roasted vegetables

For extra flavor, before grilling or roasting, marinate the vegetables for 30 minutes to 1 hour in one of these marinades:

Basic Marinade
⅛ cup reduced-sodium soy sauce
¼ cup balsamic vinegar
¼ cup extra virgin olive oil
¼ cup water
2 garlic cloves, minced
  Freshly-ground black pepper

Italian Marinade
2 tablespoons chopped fresh oregano
2 tablespoons chopped fresh basil
1 cup *Basic Marinade*

Southwestern Marinade
3-4 tablespoon chopped fresh sage
1-2 fresh/dried chili
½ cup *Basic Marinade*

Asian Marinade
⅔ cup rice vinegar
2 tablespoons lemon juice
2 tablespoons Dijon mustard
1 tablespoon toasted sesame oil
  sea salt, freshly-ground black pepper
4 garlic cloves, minced

Topping Mixes (add to vegetables after grilling or roasting)
- Chopped curly parsley, Parmesan cheese, capers, 1 tablespoon extra virgin olive oil, 1 teaspoon lemon juice

- Chopped fresh dill, shaved red onions, feta cheese, 1 teaspoon lemon juice, freshly-ground black pepper

183

basic stir-fried vegetables

Serves 4
Nutritional values vary depending on the selection and quantity of vegetables.
¼ of sauce ingredients and olive oil = 44 Calories per serving; 1g CHO; 5g FAT; 0g PRO; 0g Fiber

Sauce

⅓ cup chicken broth
1 tablespoon reduced-sodium soy sauce
½ tablespoon rice wine
1 teaspoon toasted sesame oil

Main Ingredients

1 tablespoon extra virgin olive oil
⅓ teaspoon minced gingerroot
2 garlic cloves, minced
1 pound (3-4 cups) vegetables (your choice)
1 teaspoon arrowroot
2 tablespoons cold water

Mix sauce ingredients together in a small bowl, and set aside. Prepare selected vegetables (see combinations on following page) by cutting to similar sizes to promote even cooking. In a large skillet or wok, heat olive oil over medium-high heat. Add gingerroot and garlic and stir-fry for 5-10 seconds. Add prepared vegetables, densest first (i.e., carrots), and stir-fry 3-5 minutes. Add sauce; heat through or simmer covered over medium heat until vegetables are done. Mix arrowroot and cold water together and pour over cooked vegetables.

Vegetable Combinations

- Asparagus, onions, carrot
- Bok choy, onions, carrot, mushrooms
- Broccoli, mushrooms, carrots, water chestnuts
- Broccoli, cabbage, mushrooms, carrots, onions
- Cabbage, green onions, dried shiitake mushrooms
  (soaked to soften; thinly sliced)
- Cabbage, onions, green pepper, fresh mushrooms, carrots, snow peas
- Green beans or Swiss chard
- Snow peas, julienne carrots, onion, mushrooms
- Spinach, green onions, water chestnuts
- Zucchini, green pepper, mushrooms, onions, tomatoes

Sauce Variations

- Season hot oil with 2 or more dried red chili peppers
- Add ¼ teaspoon hot chili paste to Sauce
- Add ½ tablespoon hoisin sauce to Sauce

marinated asparagus tips

Serves 6
38 Calories per serving; 6g CHO; 1g FAT; 3g PRO; 5g Fiber

2   pounds asparagus, washed and trimmed
    water
½   teaspoon sea salt
2   tablespoons lemon juice
2   garlic cloves, minced
1   tablespoon reduced-sodium soy sauce
2   tablespoons white rice vinegar
1   teaspoon toasted sesame oil

Put 2-3 inches of water in a skillet. Add sea salt and lemon juice; bring to boil. Add asparagus. Simmer covered for 2-7 minutes, depending on thickness of spears and desired crispness. Drain. Plunge cooked asparagus into cold water for 1 minute. Drain and place on layers of paper towel. Place asparagus in serving bowl. In small bowl, mix garlic, soy sauce, rice vinegar, and sesame oil. Pour over asparagus. Refrigerate for at least a few hours before serving.

green beans amandine

Serves 2
81 Calories per serving; 9g CHO; 5g FAT; 3g PRO; 4g Fiber

½   pound green beans, washed and trimmed
1   tablespoon slivered almonds
½   tablespoon butter
1   teaspoon lemon juice

Bring 1 cup of water to boil in medium saucepan. Add beans and reduce to low-medium heat. Cook beans for 5-7 minutes, drain and set aside. In medium skillet, heat butter over low-medium heat; add almonds, stirring occasionally, until golden. Remove from heat; add lemon juice. Pour over beans.

basic sautéed tender greens (beet greens, spinach, swiss chard)

Serves 4
100 Calories per serving; 10g CHO; 6g FAT; 2g PRO; 5g Fiber

2   tablespoons extra virgin olive oil
1   tablespoon garlic cloves, cut into very thin strips
1   pound fresh tender greens (about 16 cups loosely packed)
    sea salt and freshly-ground black pepper, to taste
    pinch of red pepper flakes
1   tablespoon lemon juice or balsamic vinegar

Wash greens in at least two changes of cold water. Drain. Pinch stems off spinach. Tiny beets may be left on greens. Stems of Swiss chard may be left on and chopped with the greens or cut out of the leafy portion. Coarsely chop the greens into approximately 1-inch chunks. In a large skillet over medium heat, heat olive oil and garlic together for about 2 minutes. Add greens by handfuls, using tongs to stir and coat with oil. Once all the greens have been added, sprinkle with salt, red pepper flakes, and black pepper. Continue stirring until greens are uniformly wilted and glossy (about 2 minutes). Transfer greens to a colander in the sink and gently squeeze greens with tongs to release excess juices. Return greens to the skillet; sprinkle with lemon juice or balsamic vinegar and stir to coat. Drizzle with an additional 1 teaspoon of olive oil, if desired. Serve immediately.

basic sautéed tough greens (collards, kale, mustard, turnip)

Serves 4
100 Calories per serving; 10g CHO; 6g FAT; 2g PRO; 5g Fiber

	sea salt
2	quarts water
1	pound tough greens (about 16 cups loosely packed)
1	tablespoon garlic cloves, cut into thin slices
	pinch of red pepper flakes
2	tablespoons extra virgin olive oil
⅓	cup chicken broth
1	tablespoon lemon juice or balsamic vinegar

Wash the greens in at least two changes of cold water. Drain. To remove stems, lay each leaf on a cutting board and cut out with a knife. Coarsely chop the greens into approximately 1-inch chunks. In a large pot, bring 2 quarts of water to a boil. Add 1 teaspoon sea salt and greens; stir. Cover and cook the greens for about 7 minutes. Drain in a colander in the sink. Refill the pot with cold water and add the cooked greens to stop the cooking process. Drain the greens again in the colander. In a large skillet, heat oil, garlic and red pepper flakes for about 1 minute. Add greens and stir to coat with the oil. Add broth; cover and cook over medium-high heat about 5 more minutes, until the greens are tender and juicy and most of the broth has been absorbed. Serve immediately, sprinkled with lemon juice or balsamic vinegar.

roasted sweet potato wedges

Serves 4
150 Calories per serving; 24g CHO; 5g FAT; 2g PRO; 3g Fiber

1   pound pared sweet potatoes (2 large), each cut into 8 lengthwise wedges
1½   tablespoons extra virgin olive oil
½   teaspoon sea salt

Lightly coat a cookie sheet with olive oil. Place potato wedges on cookie sheet
and sprinkle with olive oil and sea salt. Lay wedges on one cut side. Bake at 425°
for 15 minutes. Turn each wedge to its other cut side for even caramelizing,
and bake another 15 minutes. Fresh vegetables may be added to roast for the last
10-15 minutes.

roasted redskin potatoes

Serves 4
125 Calories per serving; 23g CHO; 5g FAT; 4g PRO; 2g Fiber

1	pound small redskin potatoes, scrubbed clean, dried, halved (cut into quarters if large)
1½	tablespoons extra virgin olive oil
10-12	whole garlic cloves, peeled and left whole
	sea salt and freshly-ground black pepper, to taste

Adjust oven rack to middle position and heat oven to 425°. Toss potatoes, garlic, and olive oil in medium bowl to coat. Season with salt and pepper and toss again to blend. Place potatoes flesh side down in a single layer on shallow roasting pan or cookie sheet. Roast until side of potato touching pan is crusty golden brown, about 20-30 minutes. Remove pan from oven and carefully turn potatoes over using metal spatula. Return pan to oven and roast until side of potato now touching pan is crusty golden brown and skins have raisin-like wrinkles, 5-10 minutes more. Remove from oven, transfer potatoes to serving dish and serve warm with low-fat sour cream/horseradish/chive sauce.

Variation: Sprinkle 1 pound of fresh asparagus, green beans, and/or onions with olive oil and add to the pan during the last 10-15 minutes to roast with the potatoes.

oven french fries

Serves 4
125 Calories per serving; 23g CHO; 5g FAT; 4g PRO; 2g Fiber

1	pound large redskin potatoes, scrubbed clean, dried, cut into shoestrings
1½	tablespoons extra virgin olive oil
	sea salt and freshly-ground black pepper, to taste

Adjust oven rack to middle position and heat oven to 425°. Toss potatoes and olive oil on cookie sheet; season with salt and pepper and toss again to blend. Spread potatoes out in a single layer. Cook for 15 minutes; turn French fries over using metal spatula. Return pan to oven and cook 10-15 minutes more until the potatoes begin to get browned and crunchy.

mama DeRose's tomatoes

per Patricia DeRose Lewis
Serves 4
81 Calories per serving; 10g CHO; 5g FAT; 1g PRO; 2g Fiber

1	room temperature green pepper, sliced
3-4	room temperature tomatoes, sliced
1-2	onions, sliced

Place sliced vegetables in a bowl, sprinkle with sea salt and drizzle with extra virgin olive oil. Let set 10 minutes. Gobble up. Don't refrigerate!!! Also very good with a room temperature, peeled cucumber sliced into it.

fresh tomato salad

4 cups
I cup = 82 Calories; 12g CHO; 4g FAT; 2g PRO; 3g Fiber

4   cups unpeeled tomatoes, cut in bite-size pieces
¼   cup Italian flat leaf parsley, chopped
I   tablespoon red wine vinegar
I   teaspoon Dijon mustard
I   tablespoon extra virgin olive oil
I   garlic clove, minced
    sea salt and freshly-ground black pepper, to taste

Toss all ingredients together and let marinate 1 hour or longer before serving.

🌀 greek tomato salad

6 cups
1 cup = 103 Calories; 12g CHO; 6g FAT; 3g PRO; 3g Fiber

¼ cup red wine vinegar
2 tablespoons extra virgin olive oil
2 garlic cloves, minced
½ teaspoon dried oregano
¼ teaspoon dried basil
  sea salt and freshly-ground black pepper, to taste
1 cup thinly sliced red onion, rings quartered
1 green pepper, cut in 1-inch chunks
6 medium unpeeled tomatoes, each cut into 8 wedges, then halved
6 medium pitted whole ripe olives, halved
3 tablespoons crumbled feta cheese

In a medium bowl, whisk together vinegar, olive oil, garlic, oregano, basil, salt and pepper. Add prepared vegetables, olives and cheese. Cover and let sit on the counter for at least 1 hour to season; stir occasionally to blend flavors. Great on bed of Romaine lettuce. Refrigerate leftovers.

Variation: Add 12 spears of asparagus which have been cut into 1-inch pieces, steamed, placed in ice water to prevent further cooking, and drained.

VEGETABLES AND SIDES

193

tomato salsa (mild)

5 cups
½ cup = 37 Calories; 6g CHO; 2g FAT; 1g PRO; 2g Fiber

3   cups fresh tomatoes, peeled, seeded, minced and drained
½   cup minced onion
½   cup minced celery
½   cup minced green pepper
2   tablespoons red wine vinegar
1   tablespoon extra virgin olive oil
2   garlic cloves, minced
½   teaspoon dried cilantro
1   teaspoon cumin
½   teaspoon dried sweet basil
1   teaspoon sea salt
2   4-ounce cans green chilies, chopped

Combine all ingredients in a medium bowl and blend well. Cover and chill several hours or overnight. Can be used in many ways, including: served with blue corn chips as a snack, used as a ketchup replacement, added to soups or scrambled eggs, or as a spread on meatloaf.

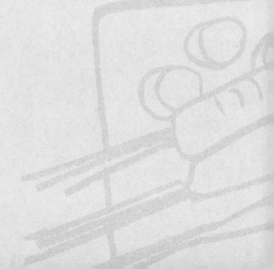

vegetable-tomato sauce

6 cups
1½ cups = 119 Calories; 15g CHO; 3g FAT; 8g PRO; 7g Fiber (not including potatoes or pasta)

1	tablespoon extra virgin olive oil
1	medium onion, chopped
1	pound mushrooms, sliced
1-2	garlic cloves, minced
1	red bell pepper, chopped
2	small zucchini, sliced
1	28-ounce can tomato sauce
¼	cup Italian flat-leaf parsley, chopped
1	teaspoon fresh chopped oregano
	sea salt and freshly-ground black pepper, to taste
1½	tablespoons fresh basil, chopped
1	cup kale or spinach, chopped

Heat olive oil in large skillet; sauté onion, mushrooms, bell pepper and garlic for 5 minutes. Add zucchini, tomato sauce, parsley, oregano, sea salt and freshly-ground black pepper to taste. Cook uncovered for 1 hour over medium-low heat, stirring occasionally. Stir in basil and kale or spinach. Cook just until greens wilt, 2-3 minutes. Serve over baked redskin potatoes or whole grain pasta.

VEGETABLES AND SIDES

195

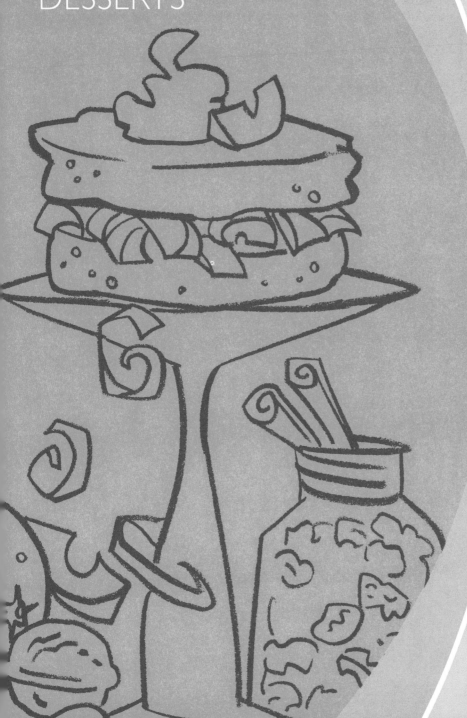

DESSERTS

desserts

🍭 = Cook's Favorite

fruit gelatin

4 cups
½ cup = 78 Calories; 17g CHO; 0g Fat; 1g PRO; 2g Fiber

2   cups unsweetened 100% fruit juice
1   teaspoon agar powder
1   teaspoon Stevia Plus™ blend
2   oranges, peeled and sliced
2   bananas, peeled and sliced

Pour juice in a medium saucepan and sprinkle agar powder over the juice. Bring to a gentle boil and cook for 1 minute. Remove pan from heat. Stir in Stevia Plus™. Let mixture cool for 1 minute. Add prepared fruits, pour into serving bowl and refrigerate to complete setting, about 30 minutes to 1 hour.

crustless pumpkin pie

Serves 8
69 Calories per serving; 12g CHO; < .5g FAT; 6g PRO; 3g Fiber

1	teaspoon extra virgin coconut oil
5	teaspoons Stevia Plus™ blend
2	tablespoons water
4	egg whites (free-range), slightly beaten
1	12-ounce can organic, fat-free evaporated milk
2	tablespoons unsweetened natural applesauce
¼	teaspoon ground nutmeg
1½	teaspoons cinnamon
½	teaspoon ground ginger
¼	teaspoon cloves
½	teaspoon sea salt
2	teaspoons vanilla extract
1	15-ounce can pumpkin

Preheat oven to 350°. Brush a 9- or 10-inch pie pan with oil. In a medium bowl, stir Stevia Plus™ into water until dissolved. (Omit the water if you use sugar instead of stevia.) Add remaining ingredients to bowl in order listed, stirring after each addition, and whisk together until well blended. Pour into pan and bake for 50-55 minutes or until knife inserted in center comes out clean.

chocolate pie (or pudding)

8 servings, ½ cup each

254 Calories per serving; 49g CHO; 3g FAT; 6g PRO; < 1g Fiber (with sugar, not including crust)

177 Calories per serving; 30g CHO; 3g FAT; 6g PRO; < 1g Fiber (with half sugar and half Stevia Plus™, not including crust)

99 Calories per serving; 10g CHO; 3g FAT; 6g PRO; < 1g Fiber (with no sugar, Stevia Plus™ only, not including crust)

The amount of sugar makes a big difference in the number of carbohydrate grams and "empty" calories in any recipe. The options are all listed here, so you can make an informed choice when making this yummy dessert.

3	cups soy milk
1½	cups granulated sugar (OR ¾ cup sugar + 3 tablespoons Stevia Plus™ blend; OR 6 tablespoons Stevia Plus™)
5	tablespoons arrowroot
½	teaspoon sea salt
½	cup unsweetened cocoa powder
4	eggs (free-range)
1	teaspoon vanilla extract
1	9-inch **Chocolate-Crumb Pie Crust** (p 202)

Combine milk, sugar and/or Stevia Plus™, arrowroot and salt in medium saucepan and whisk. Bring to near boil and whisk in cocoa. Reduce heat and simmer for 5 minutes, whisking frequently, until mixture thickens. In medium bowl, beat eggs and *very slowly* add 1 cup of the cocoa mixture, whisking constantly so the eggs don't scramble. Return this egg and cocoa mixture to the saucepan. Increase heat, bring to a boil and cook, stirring constantly for 1 minute. Remove from heat and stir in vanilla. Let cool for 2 minutes. Pour chocolate mixture into chilled *Chocolate Crumb Pie Crust* and cover with a sheet of waxed paper. Refrigerate 4 hours. Serve chilled; may be cut into individual serving sizes and frozen, then thawed when ready to serve. (For pudding, make same as above, but pour into 8 individual serving bowls, cover with plastic wrap and refrigerate 3-4 hours.)

chocolate-crumb pie crust

One 9-inch crust - Serves 8
170 Calories per serving; 22g CHO; 8g FAT; 2g PRO; 1g Fiber

1	teaspoon extra virgin coconut oil
3	tablespoons butter
1	ounce bittersweet chocolate, chopped
45	chocolate wafers (8 ounces)

Lightly coat a 9-inch glass pie pan with coconut oil. In small saucepan, combine butter and chocolate and melt over low heat, stirring frequently. Finely grind cookies in food processor. Add chocolate mixture and process again until crumbs are just moistened. Press crumb mixture along bottom and sides of pie pan. Freeze for at least 30 minutes before filling.

pumpkin cookies

36 cookies
71 Calories per serving; 12g CHO; 3g FAT; 1g PRO; 1g Fiber

1	cup packed light brown sugar
⅓	cup almond oil
1	cup canned solid pack pumpkin
1	teaspoon vanilla extract
1½	cups white whole wheat flour (unbleached, unbromated)
½	teaspoon aluminum-free baking powder
½	teaspoon baking soda
1	teaspoon cinnamon
½	teaspoon allspice
½	teaspoon sea salt
½	cup dates, chopped
½	cup hulled, coarsely-chopped pumpkin seeds

Preheat oven to 350°. In a large bowl, combine sugar and oil. Beat with electric mixer on medium speed until well blended. Mix in pumpkin and vanilla until well blended, scraping down sides of bowl as needed. On low speed, beat in all remaining ingredients except dates and pumpkin seeds. Stir in pumpkin seeds and dates by hand. Drop dough by rounded teaspoonfuls, 2 inches apart, onto an oiled cookie sheet. Using a fork, press cookies to flatten slightly. Bake on middle rack of oven until lightly browned, about 11-12 minutes. Transfer cookies to wire rack to cool. Can be frozen.

cookies that "rock"

48 cookies
89 Calories per serving; 11g CHO; 4g FAT; 3g PRO 1g Fiber (with sugar)
72 Calories per serving; 7g CHO; 4g FAT; 3g PRO; 1g Fiber (with Stevia Plus™)

1	cup whole wheat flour (unbleached, unbromated)
1	cup rolled oats
¾	cup ground flaxseeds
1	teaspoon cinnamon
1	teaspoon baking soda
1	teaspoon sea salt
1	cup whey protein powder
1	cup packed brown sugar (OR 4 tablespoons Stevia Plus™ blend)
6	egg whites (free-range)
½	cup natural unsweetened applesauce
1	teaspoon almond oil
1	tablespoon vanilla extract
1	cup chocolate chips
¾	cup chopped walnuts

Preheat oven to 350°. Combine dry ingredients, except chocolate chips and nuts, and mix well. Add egg whites, applesauce, oil and vanilla. Beat with electric mixer until combined. Stir in chocolate chips and nuts. For each cookie, drop 1 rounded teaspoon of dough onto oiled cookie sheet, 2 inches apart, flattening slightly. Bake on middle rack of oven for 6-7 minutes (for soft cookie) to 10 minutes (for crunchy cookie). Transfer cookies to a wire rack to cool. Can be frozen.

chocolate protein brownies

Serves 16
95 Calories per serving; 13g CHO; 3g FAT; 4g PRO; < 1g Fiber

½   cup natural soy protein powder
½   cup granulated sugar
5   tablespoons unsweetened cocoa powder
¾   cup white whole wheat flour (unbleached, unbromated)
¼   teaspoon sea salt
¼   teaspoon cinnamon
¾   teaspoon baking soda
¾   cup warm water
1   teaspoon vanilla extract
2   tablespoon extra virgin coconut oil, melted
2   teaspoons apple cider vinegar
2   egg whites or 1 whole egg (free-range)
2   tablespoons chopped walnuts (optional)

Preheat oven to 350°. Lightly coat the inside of an 8x8-inch baking pan with extra virgin coconut oil. Measure dry ingredients into medium bowl and mix well. Add warm water, vanilla, oil, vinegar and egg white. Stir until combined. Spread batter into baking pan and sprinkle with nuts. Bake 18-20 minutes.

carrot cake

Serves 8
283 Calories per serving; 33g CHO; 13g FAT; 8g PRO; 5g Fiber (with sugar)
253 Calories per serving; 26g CHO; 13g FAT; 8g PRO; 5g Fiber (with sugar and Stevia Plus™)

2   tablespoons extra virgin coconut oil, softened
2   eggs (free-range)
¾   cup granulated sugar (OR ⅓ cup sugar + 1½ tablespoons Stevia Plus™ blend)
¼   cup skim milk
½   teaspoon vanilla extract
1   tablespoon cinnamon
½   teaspoon ground nutmeg
1⅓ cups white whole wheat flour (unbleached, unbromated)
½   cup ground flaxseeds, flax meal or chopped walnuts
1   teaspoon baking soda
1   teaspoon aluminum-free baking powder
½   teaspoon sea salt
1½ cups grated carrots
½   cup raisins
1   teaspoon orange peel, grated

Preheat oven to 350°. In a large bowl, beat oil, eggs, sugar (and Stevia Plus™, if used), milk and vanilla with a mixer (or by hand) until creamy. Mix cinnamon, nutmeg, flour, flax (or walnuts, if used), baking soda, baking powder and salt in a separate bowl; then add to the egg mixture. Beat for an additional minute. Add carrots, raisins and orange peel; stir until combined. Spoon batter into a lightly oiled 8x8-inch baking pan and bake 30-40 minutes or until done. Cake is done when you touch it lightly in the center, and it springs back.

hazelnut fudge cake

Serves 12
226 Calories per serving; 35g CHO; 7g FAT; 5g PRO; 3g Fiber (with sugar)
161 Calories per serving; 18g CHO; 7g FAT; 5g PRO; 3g Fiber (with Stevia Plus™)

1	cup chopped pitted prunes
⅓	cup apple juice
1½	cups soy milk
5	eggs (free-range)
2	teaspoons vanilla extract
1¼	cups unsweetened cocoa powder
1	cup granulated sugar (OR 4 tablespoons Stevia Plus™ blend)
2	cups white whole wheat flour (unbleached, unbromated)
2	teaspoons aluminum-free baking powder
½	cup coarsely-ground hazelnuts

Preheat oven to 350°. Coat 9-inch spring form pan with extra virgin coconut oil. In small saucepan, combine prunes and apple juice. Bring to a boil, reduce heat and simmer uncovered 5-7 minutes or until prunes are soft. Transfer to a food processor and puree to a paste. Add milk and pulse 4-5 times. Add eggs and vanilla and pulse an additional 4-5 times. In large bowl, combine cocoa, sugar (or Stevia Plus™), flour and baking powder. Add prune/egg mixture to dry ingredients in large bowl and stir just until combined. Mix in hazelnuts. Pour batter into oiled spring form pan and bake 40-45 minutes, or until a toothpick inserted in center comes out with moist crumbs attached. Let cool 10 minutes before removing ring. Freezes well. Very chocolaty!

apple crisp

Serves 8
200 Calories per serving; 28g CHO; 8g FAT; 4g PRO; 9g Fiber

5 pounds apples, peeled and sliced
2 teaspoons cinnamon
2 cups rolled oats
1 cup whole wheat flour (unbleached, unbromated)
¼ cup packed brown sugar
¼ teaspoon sea salt
1 teaspoon aluminum-free baking powder
2 eggs (free range)
½ cup butter, melted

Preheat oven to 325°. Toss apples with cinnamon and arrange in bottom of a 9x13-inch pan. In a medium bowl, mix dry ingredients together. In a small bowl, lightly beat eggs. Add eggs to dry ingredients and gently work in eggs until mixture is crumbly. Sprinkle mixture on top of apples. Pour melted butter evenly over the top. Bake 1 hour.

blueberry cobbler

Serves 9
146 Calories per serving; 28g CHO; 5g FAT; 2g PRO; 6g Fiber

 5 cups fresh or frozen blueberries
 3 tablespoons sugar
 2 tablespoons Stevia Plus™ blend
1½ tablespoons arrowroot
 1 tablespoon lemon juice
    dash of cinnamon
 ¾ cup *Whole Grain Baking Mix* (p 52)
 ⅓ cup soy milk
 3 tablespoons extra virgin coconut oil, melted

Pour blueberries in an 8x8-inch glass baking dish. Sprinkle with sugar,
Stevia Plus™, arrowroot, lemon juice and cinnamon and stir with a fork. Preheat
oven to 400°and put blueberry mixture in oven while it is preheating. In a small
bowl, combine baking mix, milk and coconut oil; mix well with a fork. (Batter
will harden when the oil is added, no problem!) Remove pan of blueberries from
oven, and drop batter by spoonfuls on top of blueberries. Return pan to oven and
bake for 30 minutes until biscuits are slightly browned.

APPENDICES

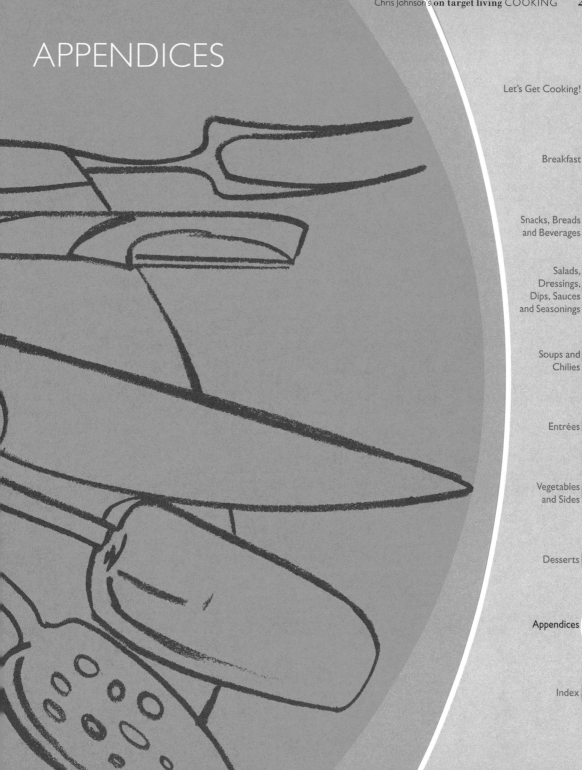

appendices

equipment list

Pots and Pans

Skillets or sauté pans with covers: 8-inch and 10-inch (or 12-inch)

Saucepans with covers: 1-quart, 2-quart, 4-quart

Stockpot or spaghetti cooker: 12- to 16-quart

Rimmed cookie sheet or shallow roasting pan

Pie pan, 9-inch, preferably glass

Bread pan, 9 x 4 inch

Cake pans, preferably glass: 8-inch square, 9-inch square, 9x13-inch

1½-quart covered casserole

Mixing bowls, stainless steel or glass: small, medium, large

Wire cooling rack

Utensils

Paring knife

Chef's knife

Vegetable peeler

Cutting board

Can opener

Measuring cups and spoons

Rubber spatula

Metal spatula

Spoons, metal and wooden

Metal meat tenderizer

Wire whisk

Potato masher

Metal or bamboo kebab skewers

Strainer/Colander

Vegetable steaming rack

equipment list

Appliances

    Stove with oven

    Blender

Miscellaneous

    Paper towels

    Plastic wrap

    Aluminum foil

    Zip top bags

Helpful but not required

    Food processor

    Mini-Mate Quisinart™ or coffee grinder

    Gas or charcoal outdoor grill; electric indoor grill

on target living nutrition shopping list

CARBOHYDRATES

Vegetables (fresh or frozen except where noted)
❏ alfalfa sprouts
❏ artichoke hearts
❏ asparagus
❏ avocadoes
❏ barley sprouts
❏ bean sprouts
❏ beans, green
❏ beets
❏ bok choy
❏ broccoli
❏ broccoli slaw
❏ Brussels sprouts
❏ cabbage
❏ carrots
❏ cauliflower
❏ celery
❏ chilies, green (canned)
❏ corn
❏ cucumber
❏ eggplant
❏ garlic
❏ leeks
❏ mushrooms (button, crimini, Portobello, shiitake)
❏ onions (dried, green [scallions], red, yellow)
❏ parsley, Italian flat leaf
❏ parsnips
❏ peas, green (frozen)
❏ peppers (red, green, yellow, jalapeño)
❏ pickle, dill
❏ potatoes (purple, redskin and sweet)
❏ pumpkin (canned)
❏ radish
❏ rutabaga
❏ salad greens (arugula, Bibb lettuce, Romaine lettuce, watercress)
❏ snow pea pods
❏ squash, winter (butternut, acorn)
❏ tender greens (beet, spinach, Swiss chard)
❏ tough greens (collards, kale, mustard, turnip)
❏ tomatoes (fresh, canned Italian stewed, paste, pizza sauce, puree, salsa, sauce, spaghetti sauce, juice)
❏ vegetable blend juice, low-sodium
❏ water chestnuts (canned)
❏ zucchini

Fruits (fresh or frozen except where noted)
❏ apples (fresh, dried, cider, juice)
❏ applesauce, unsweetened natural (canned)
❏ apricots (dried)
❏ banana
❏ blueberries (fresh or frozen)
❏ cherries (dried, fresh, frozen)
❏ cranberries (dried)
❏ cranberry juice
❏ dates (dried)
❏ grapes (red and green)
❏ kiwi
❏ lemons (for zest and juice)
❏ lime (for zest and juice)
❏ mandarin oranges (canned)
❏ mango
❏ oranges
❏ orange juice
❏ peaches
❏ pears
❏ pineapple (fresh, canned)
❏ pomegranate juice
❏ prunes (dried)
❏ raisins (dried)
❏ red raspberries
❏ strawberries (fresh, frozen)

Cereals/Breads/Grains
❏ barley, pearled
❏ breads (buns/rolls, lavash, pita, pizza crust, whole wheat, sprouted grain)
❏ bulgur
❏ cereal, Ezekiel 4:0 Original™
❏ cereal, Uncle Sam™
❏ cookies, chocolate wafer, natural
❏ cornmeal
❏ flour, whole grain unbleached, unbromated (wheat, rice, oat…)*
❏ noodles, whole grain
❏ oat bran
❏ oats, rolled
❏ pasta, whole grain (capellini, couscous, lasagna, macaroni, noodles, penne, spaghetti, vermicelli …)
❏ quinoa
❏ rice, brown, long-grain
❏ rice, mixed wild
❏ rice cakes, whole grain
❏ rice protein powder
❏ tortilla chips (high-oleic safflower oil or expeller pressed canola oil)
❏ Wasa™ crackers
❏ wheat gluten

Beans/Legumes
❏ beans (black, cannellini, garbanzo, great northern, kidney, navy, pinto, red, refried [fat-free, canned], white)
❏ hummus (prepared)
❏ lentils

PROTEINS

Meat/Poultry/Fish
❏ beef (sirloin, tenderloin, flank steak)
❏ buffalo (ground, medallions, roast, steak)
❏ chicken breast, boneless/ skinless
❏ chicken thighs (bone-in, boneless)
❏ clams (canned)
❏ cod, wild-caught
❏ crab
❏ ostrich, ground
❏ pork (loin chops, tenderloin)
❏ red snapper
❏ salmon, wild-caught
❏ scallops
❏ shrimp
❏ tuna fish, wild-caught (canned in water)
❏ turkey (ground breast, whole, ham [uncured, nitrate and nitrite-free], deli slices)
❏ venison, ground, steaks

on target living nutrition shopping list

Eggs/Dairy
- ❏ butter, organic
- ❏ cheese, organic, low-fat (cheddar, cottage, feta, pepper, Monterey jack, mozzarella, ricotta, swiss, Parmesan)
- ❏ cream, sour (organic, low-fat)
- ❏ eggs, organic, free-range
- ❏ goatein powder
- ❏ milk , organic (canned fat-free evaporated, non-fat dry powder, skim [almond, goat, oat or rice milk can be substituted in recipes for cow=s milk])
- ❏ whey protein powder
- ❏ yogurt, organic, low-fat (plain and flavored)

Soy
- ❏ milk, soy
- ❏ milk, soy (carob)
- ❏ soy meat substitute
- ❏ soy protein powder
- ❏ Soy Delicious Frozen Dessert] (chocolate velvet)
- ❏ tofu, firm

FATS (unrefined)
Nuts and Seeds
- ❏ almond butter*
- ❏ almonds, raw (sliced or slivered)
- ❏ Brazil nuts
- ❏ flax meal*
- ❏ flaxseeds, whole
- ❏ hazelnuts
- ❏ peanut butter, natural (smooth or crunchy*
- ❏ peanuts
- ❏ pine nuts
- ❏ pumpkin seeds
- ❏ sunflower seeds
- ❏ walnuts*

Oils
- ❏ almond oil
- ❏ canola oil, expeller pressed
- ❏ canola oil mayonnaise
- ❏ coconut oil, extra virgin, unrefined
- ❏ cod liver oil, lemon-flavored
- ❏ Earth Balance] spread*

- ❏ flaxseed oil*
- ❏ macadamia nut oil
- ❏ olive oil, extra virgin, unrefined
- ❏ sesame oil, toasted*

Other
- ❏ **avocado**
- ❏ **olives, green and ripe**

HERBS/SPICES/ CONDIMENTS
- ❏ allspice
- ❏ anchovy paste
- ❏ barbecue sauce
- ❏ basil, sweet (dried or fresh)
- ❏ bay leaves (dried)
- ❏ Bragg Liquid Aminos™
- ❏ capers
- ❏ chili powder
- ❏ chives ,fresh
- ❏ cilantro
- ❏ cinnamon (ground, stick)
- ❏ cloves
- ❏ coriander
- ❏ cumin, ground
- ❏ dill (dried or fresh)
- ❏ garlic powder
- ❏ ginger
- ❏ gingerroot (fresh)
- ❏ hoisin sauce
- ❏ horseradish
- ❏ hot pepper sauce
- ❏ Italian herb mix
- ❏ lemon pepper
- ❏ marjoram (dried or fresh)
- ❏ mint, fresh
- ❏ mustard (regular, Dijon and dry)
- ❏ nutmeg, ground
- ❏ onion powder
- ❏ oregano (dried or fresh)
- ❏ oyster sauce
- ❏ paprika
- ❏ parsley, Italian flat leaf
- ❏ peach chutney
- ❏ pepper, cayenne
- ❏ pepper, red (flakes)
- ❏ pepper, black (peppercorns)
- ❏ poultry seasoning
- ❏ rosemary

- ❏ rum extract
- ❏ sage
- ❏ savory (dried)
- ❏ sea salt
- ❏ sea salt based seasoning salt
- ❏ shoyu sauce
- ❏ soy sauce, reduced-sodium
- ❏ steak sauce, organic
- ❏ stir-fry sauce
- ❏ tamari sauce
- ❏ tarragon
- ❏ teriyaki sauce
- ❏ thyme (dried or fresh)
- ❏ vanilla extract, pure
- ❏ wine (dry white, rice)
- ❏ Worcestershire sauce

MISCELLANEOUS
- ❏ agar powder
- ❏ arrowroot
- ❏ baking powder, aluminum-free
- ❏ baking soda
- ❏ bouillon, chicken, low-sodium
- ❏ broth, low-sodium (beef, chicken, fish, vegetable)
- ❏ chocolate, bittersweet baking
- ❏ chocolate chips, organic
- ❏ cocoa powder, unsweetened
- ❏ maple syrup
- ❏ sweeteners (honey, Stevia Plus™ blend, brown and granulated sugar)
- ❏ vinegars (balsamic, apple cider, red wine, rice, tarragon)
- ❏ water (filtered, still and carbonated mineral)

* Store whole grain flours, unrefined oils, ground flaxseeds and raw nuts in refrigerator to protect against rancidity and nutrient loss. Whole grain flours can also be frozen to protect freshness.

menu plans for weeks 1 and 2

MENU FOR WEEK 1

DAY	BREAKFAST	SNACK	LUNCH	SNACK	DINNER
1	*Asparagus Quiche* Whole grain toast	Yogurt, mixed fruit, flaxseed oil or flavored cod liver oil	*Southwestern Bean Soup* ¼ avocado	Apple Peanut butter	*Pan-Seared Salmon* Tossed salad with *Greek Salad Dressing* Steamed mixed vegetables
2	*CJ's Oatmeal On-The-Run*	Apple Peanut butter	*Salmon Salad* (use leftover salmon from Day 1)	*Basic Smoothie* with blueberries	*Sloppy Joes* Whole grain roll *Fruit Gelatin*
3	Granola Bar Peanut butter Skim or soy milk	Yogurt, mixed fruit, flaxseed oil or flavored cod liver oil	*Southwestern Bean Soup* (leftover from Day 1)	*CJ's Granola* Almonds	*Pan-Seared Chicken Roasted Sweet Potato Wedges Basic Roasted Vegetables*
4	*Basic Smoothie* with raspberries	*Parfait On-the-Run*	*Chicken Caesar Salad* leftover chicken from Day 3	Boiled egg, carrots, celery	*Zucchini "Pasta" Pita Garlic Bread* Tossed salad with *So Simple Salad Dressing*
5	*3-Minute Scrambled Eggs* Whole grain toast Fruit	Grapes, walnuts	*Salad in a Bag* with chicken left over from Day 3	*Flax Bran Muffin* Peanut butter	*Pita Pizza* Tossed salad with *So Simple Salad Dressing*
6	*Parfait on-the-Run*	Boiled egg, banana	*Stuffed Pita* with leftover vegetables from Day 5	Almonds, grapes	*Parmesan Cod Oven French Fries Basic Sautéed Tender Greens Tartar Sauce II*
7	*Blender Breakfast*	Low-fat cottage cheese, pineapple, almonds	*Clam Chowder* Whole grain crackers	Apple Peanut butter	*Chicken Stir-Fry Basic Fried Rice*

Recipes in bold italics are included in this book.

Specific quantities are not included, as this will vary for each individual. Be sure to add ground flaxseed (or flaxseed oil) and cod liver oil each day if they are not already included in the recipes.

These sample menu plans are designed to give you a variety of options to choose from. Once you find a recipe you enjoy, feel free to repeat as needed.

menu plans for weeks 1 and 2

MENU FOR WEEK 2

DAY	BREAKFAST	SNACK	LUNCH	SNACK	DINNER
1	*Quiche* Whole grain toast	Apple Peanut butter	*Clam Chowder* leftover from Week 1, Day 7 Whole grain crackers	Yogurt, mixed fruit, flaxseed oil or flavored cod liver oil	*Buffalo Turkey Meatloaf* Baked sweet potato Tossed salad with *Caesar Salad Dressing*
2	*Breakfast Sandwich* Milk	Orange Slivered almonds	*Buffalo Turkey Meatloaf* sandwich with whole grain bread, mustard, onion, salsa	*Berry Blast Smoothie*	*Oven-Fried Chicken Basic Stir-Fried Vegetables*
3	*Creamy Oatmeal*	Milk, blueberries, almonds	Egg Salad Sandwich with whole grain bread, canola mayo, mustard	Apple Peanut butter	*Salmon Fillet in Garlic Green Beans Amandine*
4	*Scrambled Eggs* Salsa Whole grain toast	*Parfait on-the-Run*	*CJ's Big Salad* with leftover salmon from Day 3	*Turkey Roll-up*	*Easy Cookie Sheet Dinner* (with sweet potatoes and vegetables of choice)
5	*CJ's Granola* Milk Fruit	Boiled egg orange	*Cherry Chicken Salad* with leftover chicken from Day 4	Trail Mix 5 almonds	*Fast Chili* Avocado slices *Carrot Cake*
6	*Egg White Omelet* Whole grain toast	Whole grain cracker, extra virgin coconut oil, fruit spread	*Fast Chili* left over from Day 5 ¼ sliced avocado	Yogurt, fruit, flaxseed oil or flavored cod liver oil	*Carol's Pineapple Chicken* Tossed salad with *So Simple Salad Dressing*
7	*Power Pancakes*	Tuna, canola mayo, onion, chopped on celery sticks	Whole grain tortilla roll-up with hummus, mujadrah, tomato, Romaine,	*CJ's Smoothie*	*Barbecued Pork Tenderloin Basic Grilled Vegetables* Steamed Brown Rice

herbs and spices

There are hundreds of herbs, spices and blends that can enhance the flavor of foods and decrease the need to use even sea salt as a flavoring. Here are just a few.

HERBS

Dominant-flavored herbs are very potent and can be cooked for long periods of time without losing their flavor. Generally, use about 1 teaspoon of dried herb or 1 tablespoon of fresh herb to flavor 6 servings of a dish, then adjust the amount to suit your taste. These herbs can be added at the beginning of cooking your recipe.

HERB	USES
Bay leaves	Use whole and remove from the dish before serving. Use in stews, tomato sauces, soups, poaching fish, game dishes, marinades.
Black pepper	Freshly-ground, this herb enhances so many dishes.
Garlic	Oriental, Latino, Italian, Greek cuisines. Use in soups, salads, bean dishes, pesto, roasted with vegetables, chicken, sautéed in stir-fries, raw in salads or rubbed over bread with tomato and extra virgin olive oil.
Horseradish	Usually used fresh, raw. Sauces, beef, oily fish, smoked fish.
Oregano, Greek	Greek, Italian, Mexican cuisines. Use in tomato sauces, salads, pizza, pasta sauces, lamb stews, chicken, beans, game.
Rosemary	Vegetables (eggplant, beans, cabbage, zucchini, potatoes, tomatoes), roasting chicken, oily fish, marinades for game.
Sage	Stuffing, soups, sauces, vegetables, egg dishes, fish, game, beans, rice.
Stevia	Stable to 390°; sold as a dietary supplement in health food stores in powder, liquid and leaf form. Use ¼ teaspoon of powder blend to equal the sweetening effect of 1 teaspoon sugar. Vanilla extract enhances the sweetness of stevia.

herbs and spices

Medium-flavored herbs are generally less potent and maintain their full flavor for less cooking time. Use 1-2 teaspoons of the dried herb or 1-2 tablespoons of the fresh herb to flavor 6 servings of a dish, adjusting the amount to suit your taste. To maintain maximum flavor, add these herbs 5-10 minutes before the end of cooking time.

HERB	USES
Cilantro	Mexican, Chinese, Indian, Middle Eastern, Spanish cuisines. Use in combination with garlic, basil, mint, parsley, lemon and lime, chilies, coconut. Use with bean/rice dishes, fish and seafood, potatoes, salsa, chili.
Dill	Vegetables, fish, bean soups.
Marjoram	Similar to but milder than oregano. Combines well with parsley and lemon thyme. Use with beef, poultry, fish, vegetables (broccoli, zucchini, mushrooms, onions. tomato), stews, sauces, soups, pasta, fish, game, meatloaf.
Savory (winter and summer)	Similar in flavor to thyme. Use with beans, poultry, game, stews.
Tarragon, French	Fish, poultry, cheese dishes, vegetables (asparagus, leeks, avocado, mushrooms, tomato salad), eggs. Use in combination with bay leaves, parsley and thyme for *bouquet garni* in beef stews and vegetable soups. Use in combination with parsley, thyme and chervil for *fines herbes* for soups, vegetables, cottage cheese.
Thyme	French, Spanish, Latino cuisines. A great all-purpose herb with many varieties. Combines well with garlic, onion, red wine, basil, bay, marjoram, parsley and savory. Use regular thyme with shellfish, game, meats, vegetables (tomatoes, mushrooms, leeks, eggplant), salads, fish, beans, soups, stews.

herbs and spices

Delicate-flavored herbs are the least potent and maintain their best flavor only if added at the very end of cooking or used raw. Use about 1 teaspoon to 3 tablespoons of the dried herb or 1 tablespoon to ½ cup of the fresh herb to flavor a 6-serving dish, and then adjust to suit your taste. Add these herbs in the last 1-2 minutes of cooking.

HERB	USES
Basil, sweet	French and Italian cuisines. Combines well with garlic, olive oil, and lemon. Use in pesto, with tomatoes, eggs, cheese dishes, fish, poultry, beans, salads, zucchini, beans, mushrooms.
Chives	Delicate onion flavor; excellent garnish. Add at the last minute to soups, scrambled eggs.
Parsley, Italian flat leaf	French, Middle Eastern, and Italian cuisines. Pesto, salads, egg dishes, soups, potatoes, tabbouleh

SPICES

The herbs listed above are often thought of as "savory" versus "sweet" while the spices used in these recipes are generally sweet—cinnamon, ginger, nutmeg. That is, they are used most often in recipes that contain sweetener—smoothies, granola bars, oatmeal, fruit, desserts.

A wonderfully-smelling spice blend to have simmering during the holidays is: 1 whole cinnamon stick, 1 teaspoon whole allspice, 1 teaspoon whole cloves, and 1 cup of water or apple cider. Simmer in a small saucepan on the stove, and add more water or cider as the liquid reduces down.

weights and measures

CUP=	FLUID OUNCES=	TABLESPOONS=	TEASPOONS
1 C	8 oz	16 Tbsp	48 tsp
¾ C	6 oz	12 Tbsp	36 tsp
⅔ C	5⅓ oz	10.6 Tbsp	32 tsp
½ C	4 oz	8 Tbsp	24 tsp
⅓ C	2⅔ oz	5.3 Tbsp	16 tsp
¼ C	2 oz	4 Tbsp	12 tsp
⅛ C	1 oz	2 Tbsp	6 tsp
1/16 C	½ oz	1 Tbsp	3 tsp

1 cup = ½ pint

2 cups = 1 pint

4 cups = 1 quart

4 quarts = 1 gallon

8 quarts = 1 peck

4 pecks = 1 bushel

1 pound = 16 ounces dry measure

1 ounce = 28.3 grams (weight) dry measure

To convert grams to ounces, multiply number of grams by 0.0353 = ounces

To convert ounces to grams, multiply number of ounces by 28.3 = grams

general substitutions

2 teaspoons arrowroot = 1 tablespoon cornstarch or 1½ tablespoon flour

2⅛ cups uncooked rice = 1 pound

1 cup uncooked rice = 2½ cups cooked rice

1 teaspoon agar powder + 2 cups fruit juice = 3-ounce package of flavored, sugared gelatin

1 teaspoon agar powder = 1 packet of unflavored gelatin

2 cups uncooked beans = 3½ cups cooked beans

3 tablespoons unsweetened cocoa + 1 tablespoon extra virgin coconut oil =
1 ounce or 1 square baking chocolate

2½ cups raisins = 1 15-ounce package

1 cup chopped nuts = ¼ pound

Soy sauce = Bragg Liquid Aminos™, shoyu sauce

Stevia Plus™ blend	=	Sugar or Splenda™
¼ teaspoon	=	1 teaspoon
1 tablespoon	=	¼ cup
2 tablespoons	=	½ cup
¼ cup	=	1 cup

4 cups shredded cheese = 1 pound

4 tablespoons shredded cheese = 1 ounce

½ cup evaporated milk + ½ cup water = 1 cup milk

1 lemon = 2½ to 3 tablespoons juice

grated peel of 1 lemon = 1½ teaspoons zest

resources/bibliography

ChrisJohnson@OnTargetLiving.com

Fife, Bruce. *The Coconut Oil Miracle*. NY: Avery Books, 2004.

Gittleman, Ann Louise. *The Fat Flush Plan*. NY: McGraw-Hill, 2002

Hyman, M.D., Mark and Mark Liponis, M.D. *Ultraprevention: The 6-week Plan that Will Keep You Healthy for Life*. NY: Atria Books, 2003

Johnson, Chris. *Meal Patterning: Developing Healthy Nutritional Patterns for a Lifetime*. Chris Johnson, LLC, 2003.

Johnson, Chris, *On Target Living Nutrition*. On Target Living, Int'l, 2007.

Kirkland, James and Tanya. *Sugar-Free Cooking with Stevia: The Naturally Sweet and Calorie-Free Herb*. Fourth edition, revised. Arlington, TX: Crystal Health Publishing, 2002.

Meyerowitz, Steve. *The Organic Food Guide: How to Shop Smarter and Eat Healthier*. Guilford, CT: The Globe Pequot Press, 2004.

Perry, Luddene and Dan Schultz. *A Field Guide to Buying Organic*. NY: Bantam Dell. 2005

Pollan, Michael. *The Omnivore's Dilemma: A Natural History of Four Meals*. NY: Penguin Press, 2006.

Schlosser, Eric and Charles Wilson. *Chew on This: Everything You Don't Want to Know About Fast Food*. NY: Houghton Mifflin Company, 2006.

Ursell, Amanda. *What Are You Really Eating?: How to Become Label Savvy*. Carlsbad, CA: Hay House, 2005.

Wood, Rebecca. *The New Whole Foods Encyclopedia*. NY: Penguin Books, 1999.

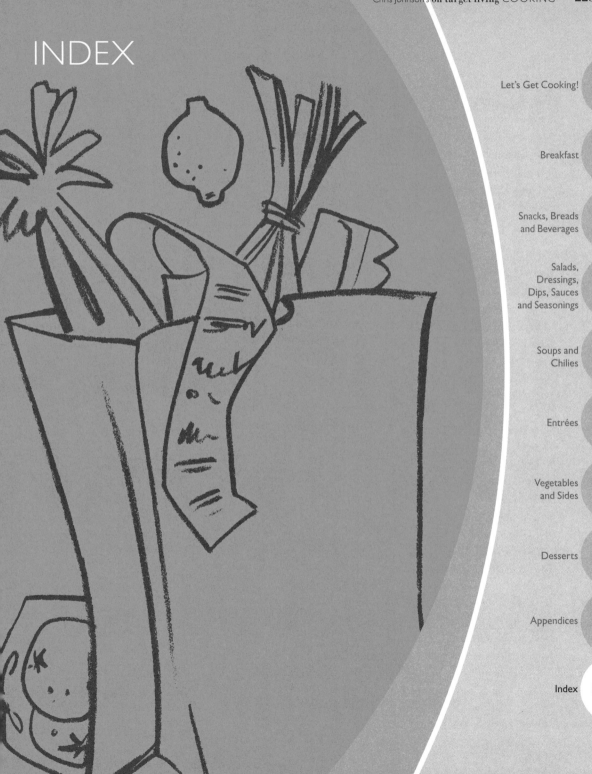

INDEX

index

index

index

index

index

index

index

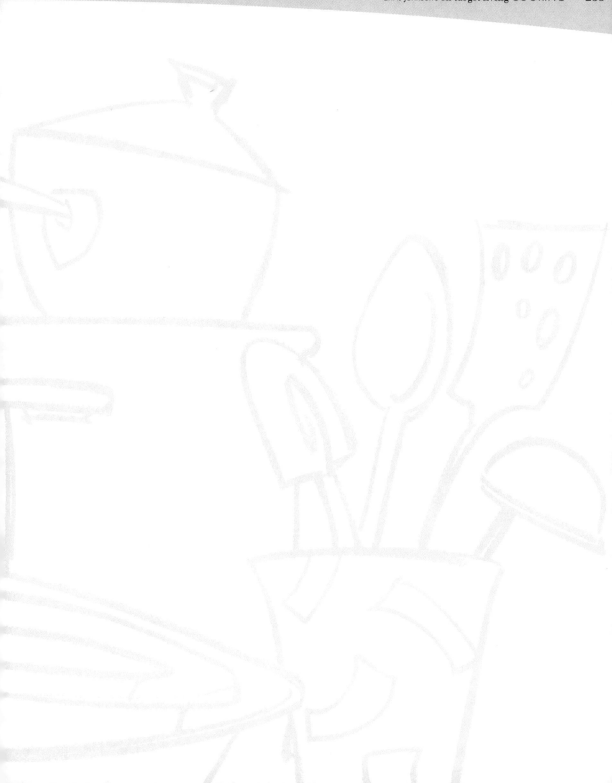

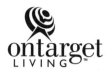

ontarget LIVING™

For more information, contact

Chris Johnson
On Target Living, Int'l
5572 Silverleaf Court
Haslett, MI 48840
(517) 339-6909
www.OnTargetLiving.com

**See the website for more information
on seminars, products and books
published by Chris Johnson**

About the authors

Chris Johnson is a nationally recognized speaker and author. For over 25 years he has earned and maintained the reputation of providing lifestyle modification strategies with integrity and compassion. Chris holds a Masters in Exercise Physiology from Michigan State University and is certified by the American College of Sports Medicine, the National Academy of Sports Medicine, and the American Council on Exercise.

Chris's mission is "to help improve the health of the United States population, one person at a time." To that end, he has developed one of the most successful club-based personal training programs in the country.

Chris lives in Haslett, Michigan, with his wife Paula, their two children, Kristen and Matt, and Dolly "The Wonder Dog."

Bonnie Klinger descends from a long line of good farm cooks who raised their own vegetables and meat, milked their own cows, made their own butter, used organic fertilizer before it was called that, and wouldn't have known a trans-fatty acid if they stepped in it. She baked her first apple pie when she was 10 years old and hasn't stopped experimenting with recipes and growing her own food since. When she's not cooking or gardening, Bonnie loves to paint (sometimes walls, sometimes pictures), read, bike, swim, do yoga, all that great exercise stuff.